T0192210

A Comprehensive Guide to Coding and Programming in Stata

This book is an introductory guide to programming and coding in Stata. It presents commonly encountered code in the field of medical statistics as well as the analyses of observational data.

For those who are involved in the analyses of observational studies, the need to sometimes assemble large datasets will necessitate a detailed understanding of loops and macros. This book covers these materials early on and then describes other commonly required coding commands.

For those who program in a controlled environment (e.g. medical statisticians who perform analyses for regulatory bodies), the production of log files, a suggested folder structure and analysis pathway are covered. This book also includes a wide range of tabulation commands and other methods of producing tables of descriptive statistics. The text also then provides a clear explanation of how to perform some inferential analyses (including how to extract and format the coefficients for use in subsequent reports).

The focus on coding allows beginners to grasp the basics of coding and programming, as well as allowing established researchers to hone their skills and become more advanced programmers.

Key features include the following:

- Covers the fundamentals of using and understanding Stata.
- Can be used by anyone looking to learn the basics of coding.
- Introduces and explains difficult concepts such as macros from the outset.

A Comprehensive Guide to Coding and Programming in Stata

Rafael Gafoor

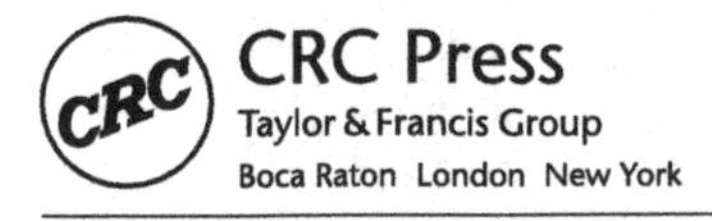

CRC Press is an imprint of the
Taylor & Francis Group, an informa business
A CHAPMAN & HALL BOOK

Designed cover image: © Shutterstock, Stock vector ID 1714491562, Vector Contributor Iurii Motov

First edition published 2024
by CRC Press
2385 NW Executive Center Drive, Suite 320, Boca Raton FL 33431

and by CRC Press
4 Park Square, Milton Park, Abingdon, Oxon, OX14 4RN

CRC Press is an imprint of Taylor & Francis Group, LLC

ISBN: 978-1-032-77485-5 (hbk)
ISBN: 978-1-032-77565-4 (pbk)
ISBN: 978-1-003-48377-9 (ebk)

DOI: 10.1201/9781003483779

Typeset in Minion
by MPS Limited, Dehradun

Contents

Foreword

THIS BOOK WAS WRITTEN AT A TIME WHEN I HAD JUST CHANGED ROLES FROM being a medical statistician (primarily concerned with the analysis of data from randomised controlled trials) to being an analyst for large datasets. I discovered that I had to learn new suites of commands in Stata and that there were advanced functions that I had never previously explored. This book comes from this experience and introduces the reader to the commands that I found the most useful. This is not to say that the commands I have chosen to explain are exhaustive in any sense of the word.

I wanted the book to be a gentle introduction to the most commonly used commands for the analyses of data obtained from both experimental as well as observational studies. I have relied on my own personal experience for guidance. No doubt you will find the book incomplete; however I hope that this guide will provide a sound platform from which you can explore further as you become an advanced Stata programmer.

This book is suitable for a wide range of professions involved in data analysis (medical statisticians, epidemiologists, data analysts, etc.).

About the Author

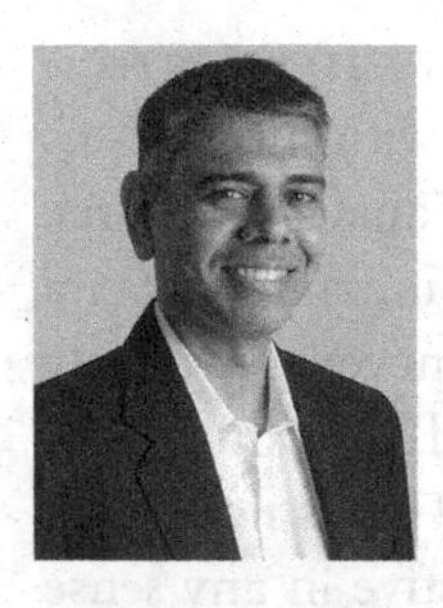

Rafael Gafoor is a Chartered Statistician at the Comprehensive Clinical Trials Unit at University College London (UCL). Dr. Gafoor obtained both his master's degrees in Epidemiology and Medical Statistics from the London School of Hygiene and Tropical Medicine and his PhD from the Institute of Psychiatry (King's College London). He has worked as a medical statistician as well as an epidemiologist. His research interests include epidemiology, clinical sciences, public health and health services and systems. Dr. Gafoor is a consultant psychiatrist in the NHS and has a keen interest in the analysis of datasets with mental health outcomes (from both observational as well as experimental studies).

CHAPTER 1

Introduction

THE PROGRAMMING ENVIRONMENT

It's important to keep a very organised programming environment and to make sure you do not EVER overwrite your primary dataset. Therefore, you should from the outset, create a directory entitled something along the lines of "Analysis Folder" and then place three folders within it.

01_Data_In
02_Programming
03_Data_Out

You can place additional folders within these folders, but this is the main structure.

NOTE: It is important to use the underscore and not leave blank spaces when programming. While leaving blank space is not necessarily an issue for Stata users in Windows, it becomes a major issue for some R commands and in other programming environments.

DATA DOWNLOAD

You should now place the files for analysis in your file named "01_Data_In". This file now should never be overwritten. Any temporary files or files which you make in the interim should now be placed in the folder named "03_Data_Out".

DOI: 10.1201/9781003483779-1

R AND STATA (FILEPATHS)

Many statisticians and data analysts program in both R and Stata. It is possible to program entirely in R, and in the future, this may be the preferable programming language. However, if you are new to analysis (and to programming) you may find it easier to start in Stata. Depending on where you study or work, you may have little choice in the program you use to analyse data. You may be working on a project that someone else has started in which case it wouldn't make much sense to start all over again and reinvent the wheel. Alternatively, you may be required to program in a given language in your workplace so as to enable more efficient working across projects.

The most pressing issue at this stage is how to write filepaths so that they can be understood in both computing environments. This is a backslash "\"; it is named because of the direction of the TOP of the hyphen with respect to the bottom. This "/" is a forward slash.

NOTE: The direction of the hyphens. Stata doesn't really care which one you use – either backslash or forward slash but R is very rigid and will only accept forward slash. The Windows operating system produces file paths using backslashes.

However, if you are going to use R and Stata simultaneously, it's better to change them as you go along to forward slashes. You can program R to accept backslashes, but it's easier at the beginning to just change the slashes so that they are in the forward direction.

CHANGING WORKING DIRECTORY

The command **pwd** will tell you where your current working directory is located.

You now need to move this working directory to the folder you created entitled **"Analysis_Folder"** or equivalent. To change the path that Stata recognises as the current working directory to match your folder location, you will use the command cd and the filepath is placed in double quotes. In the example below, the folder "Analysis_Folder" is at the root level of the C drive. You can, of course, place your folder wherever you wish and change the pathway using the "cd" command to inform Stata of the new location.

```
cd "C:/Analysis_Folder"

. cd "C:/Analysis_Folder"
C:\Analysis_Folder
```

Everything now is coded in relation to this home directory. It means that if you move the folder or send it to a colleague for further work, they only need to change one filepath, and the analysis files should work to replicate your work. This setting of the filepath is called hardcoding. This is a very important concept that you should **NEVER** hard code except at the beginning of your code and make it explicitly obvious so that it's easy for others to easily identify where code has to be amended for your analysis files to work. This hardcoding is usually placed at the top of the master file. One obvious hard code is your working directory, but there may be other occasions in which you want to use hardcoding. Do so very sparingly.

WORKING FROM YOUR HOME DIRECTORY

This home directory will become your base, and you will very rarely, if ever, move outside of this location.

One of the few instances in which you will produce output outside of the home directory is if you are the unblinded statistician in a study and you are producing output from an analysis which you do not want the blinded statistician to see. In this instance, you will hard code for the results to appear elsewhere (outside the home directory).

If, for example, you wish to create files and/or folders within your home directory, you will sometimes need to tell Stata where the home directory is. This location is stored in a macro within Stata. A macro is a piece of information which Stata stores in its memory. The different types of macros and the implications for programming will be discussed in subsequent chapters.

For example, to find a list of the files and folders within the 01_Data_In folder, you can issue the following command:

```
dir "`c(pwd)'/01_Data_In/"

<dir> 4/30/19 15:15 .
<dir> 4/30/19 15:15 ..
<dir> 4/30/19 15:15 British_Election_Survey
<dir> 1/27/19 20:07 Regional_Data
<dir> 4/30/19 15:15 Stata_Data
<dir> 4/05/19 10:07 Station_Data
<dir> 4/30/19 15:15 Tim's datasets
```

The macro 'c(pwd)' is where the contents of your working directory are stored, and you can use this as a short cut in filepaths so that you do not have to hard code again (once you have previously set the working directory). Once you set the working directory, 'c(pwd)' will always point to the correct location.

FOLDER STRUCTURE

Your coding for all projects encompasses several steps in data processing: production of interim datasets, graphs, tables, etc. If you code all of your programs for an assignment in one file, it can become very long, and you can't easily distinguish the stages in your analysis.

It is essential that you create a master file that you can use to call the subprograms from. The master file sits in the top level of the folder structure, and the subdirectories and files for your programming steps sit in the folder named "Programming". You may wish to add additional programming files in your programming folder entitled "01_Data_Input", "02_Data_Processing", "03_Tables", etc.

CREATING A "MASTER FILE"

At the root level of the analysis folder, place a Stata.do file entitled Master. This file will call all your subprograms and contains three additional crucial pieces of information.

At the top of the Master file, you should include some preliminary information about the date the file was created, the name of the programmer, the purpose of the file, the version of Stata under which it was made, the organisation to which the programmer is associated, the date on each occasion that the program was amended and the reason why, etc.

The next step is to create a section where you place all the hardcoding in your analysis. This should be the only place where hardcoding is present. This allows the analysis to very easily port across computing environments.

The next step is to place all of your global macros in a section clearly defined for this purpose. You will learn more about global macros later and the reasons why this step is so important.

The final step is to set out all of the sub-routines for your analysis so that they can be called individually and sequentially as needed.

Don't worry if this all sounds a bit complicated. It will, with time, become second nature. There will be examples of folder layouts and master files later on in the book for you to copy if you wish. Choose any file structure you wish (or adopt any you come across). The most important characteristic of a good file structure is that a reviewer should relatively easily be able to find the code, the data and the outputs without too much trouble.

SPECIAL CHARACTERS

Be sure you can identify the backtick, apostrophe, backslash, forward-slash and curly bracket characters. These will be used extensively in the course.

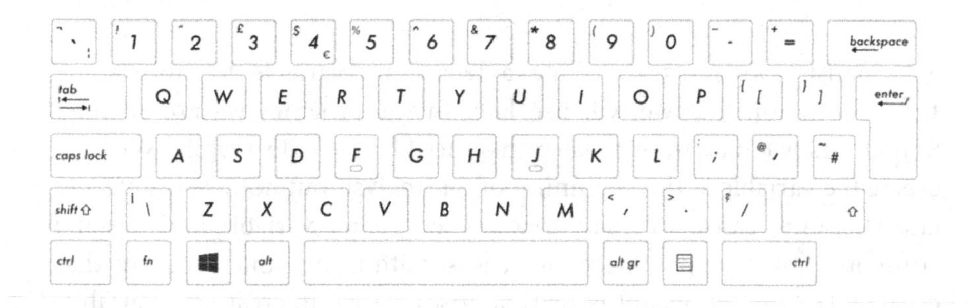

CHAPTER 2

Temporary Names, Variables and Files

Sometimes we want to create a temporary variable to store some information that we will use later in the program we are writing. Sometimes, we may want to keep this variable for quite a while. We may create the variable at the beginning of the analysis but not use it until the end. In some cases, we may create a temporary variable and use the contents almost immediately (or at least within the same program that created it). One significant issue that arises is that, in creating a variable, we might accidentally overwrite another variable with the same name. For this reason, it is good programming practice to create temporary variables with temporary names. If you keep track of these and delete them as soon as necessary, then it is less likely that you will cause errors in your analysis. Stata allows you to create three types of temporary entities – namely temporary variables, names and files. Temporary variables and names are deleted at the end of the program (environment) in which they were created, so you don't have to keep track of them once the program you have created them in has ended.

Let's imagine that I am programming an analysis for which I need to use a number which I shall call pi (persistent indigestion). This is a number to which I have assigned a value of 5.543234. Since I wish to use this number repeatedly, I wish to store it in memory so that I can easily call it into the programming environment without having to repeatedly declare it in the programming script.

DOI: 10.1201/9781003483779-2

Now, if I create a storage entity within Stata named pi, there is a chance I could start confusing this with the pi value that is already stored within Stata. Let's have a look at this first.

Let's start with an example. Stata keeps the variable pi stored as one of its inbuilt variables. We will access this using the creturn function. Don't worry about this for the moment other than to observe that Stata has a value stored within its programming environment. We will be covering creturn list later in the course. Now, let's create a value for pi (persistent indigestion), which I wish Stata to remember so that I can use it several times later in my analysis (this will reduce my workload of having to find and type in the value repeatedly, reduce the chances of errors and increase my programming efficiency). We are using a new entity (a scalar) to hold this value. Don't worry too much about this entity for the moment, we are covering this later in the course. A scalar is simply an entity that holds a single value (like a scalar in a matrix). Note that the display commands use a potentially bewildering combination of backticks, apostrophes, brackets and quotation marks. These are a source of considerable irritation and confusion to statisticians and programmers of all levels. We will be covering this syntax later in the course. For the moment, just accept they are correct.

```
display "`c(pi)'"


. display "`c(pi)'"
3.141592653589793
```

Now, generate a variable called pi with an assigned value of 87 and a scalar with a name pi and finally display all three values of "pi" that you have stored.

```
clear
scalar pi = 5.543234
set obs 20
gen pi = 87
scalar list
display scalar(pi)
display "`c(pi)'"
display pi
clear

clear
. scalar pi = 5.543234
. set obs 20
number of observations (_N) was 0, now 20
. gen pi = 87
. scalar list
      pi = 5.543234
. display scalar(pi)
5.543234
. display "`c(pi)'"
3.141592653589793
. display pi
87
. clear
```

The main take-home message is that it might be quite easy to confuse these variables and, in some environments, to overwrite them. The scalar is still in memory and will persist until you delete it.

```
scalar drop pi

scalar list
.
```

I. TEMPORARY NAMES

One way of making sure you don't overwrite existing scalars is to use a tempname. Stata keeps track of these and never uses the same name twice once you load any given name, so you needn't worry about confusing names and values. Once the program is run, and it comes to an end, the temporary entity disappears. Don't worry too much about this at this time. Just remember that you should use tempnames whenever you use a scalar. In the example below, the object is now saved as "__000001" as a temporary object in Stata, which is deleted once the program is run.

```
. tempname pi

. scalar `pi´ = 5.543234

. scalar list



. tempname pi

.
. scalar `pi' = 5.543234

.
. scalar list
  __000001 = 5.543234
```

Another commonly used method of creating a temporary entity that holds a scalar that disappears at the end of the program is to create a local. But here again you run the risk of overwriting the local (and also locals are much less efficient than scalars). I would recommend against them. We are covering locals later in this session, so no need to panic. The best solution is to use tempname in conjunction with scalars when you need to create a temporary entity that holds a single value. When you close Stata, the scalar will disappear.

A note on the naming of temporary names. You may wish to consider these as local macros. So, the syntax ` and ' that surrounds each macro is used to tell Stata that it is a macro or a scalar. You will learn more about the syntax of macros later, but it's important to realise that temporary variables are in effect local macros. Not only do they carry the syntax of a local macro, but they also disappear once used (another feature of local macros).

II. TEMPORARY VARIABLES

Now, we move on to temporary variables. If, for example, you needed to multiply every observation by a coefficient, then you could create a temporary variable. The command tempvar assigns names to the specified local macro which may then be used as a temporary variable name in a dataset.

```
tempvar coefficient

generate `coefficient' = 5.543234

display "`coefficient'"


. tempvar coefficient

.
. generate `coefficient' = 5.543234

.
. display "`coefficient'"
__000003
```

Unlike with a scalar, it is not possible to easily display the contents of a temporary variable.

Even if you had another variable called coefficient in your dataset, this would not interfere with your other variable. Stata has assigned this variable a code that **uniquely** identifies the variable and makes it impossible to confuse.

III. TEMPORARY FILES

The last of these temporary constructions is tempfile, and we will encounter this entity in more detail later in this book. Suffice to note that this creates a temporary file that but which Stata controls in such a manner that you never have to worry about them. They disappear when you close Stata, but you would never know unless you go looking for them. It's not a good idea to look for these files as some files that are not temporary and which Stata needs to work properly are very similarly named, and if you delete these files, Stata will stop running. The efficiency gained is that you end up with a clean working environment.

CHAPTER 3

Macros and Other Data Storage Mechanisms Used by Stata

I. WHERE DOES STATA STORE VARIABLES THAT YOU CANNOT READILY SEE?

Stata has multiple temporary storage features. It's best to learn about them as you need to make use of them. We will cover most (if not all) in this course. They are invaluable and are well worth the time and trouble it takes to master them. The type of storage you use depends on a number of factors:

a. Whether or not you are creating the item (or whether it is already created and stored by Stata),

b. What use will you be putting the stored item to, and

c. Whether or not it is a number.

The choices seem confusing, but as you get accustomed to programming, you will find that it becomes much easier as most people tend to use similar storage vehicles repeatedly (and they become second nature). At the beginning, they can seem confusing and a potential barrier. But having said that, you have a choice and I will give you

DOI: 10.1201/9781003483779-3

some examples of multiple ways of storing and retrieving information in Stata. Nothing is absolutely wrong (unless of course Stata throws an error), but some are more efficient in terms of time and computer resources than others. A small example would be trying to store a number in a local macro (you will learn how to do this later) rather than in a scalar. The latter is better suited, but both will work. I'll explain more about this specific example when we get to these methods of temporary data storage.

II. DEALING WITH STORAGE OF NUMBERS

a. Number Lists

The Stata command to produce a list of numbers is "numlist". This is an extremely efficient way of producing lists of numbers that you can use later (usually in a loop).

Let's enter a single number.

```
numlist "3.878"
display "`r(numlist)'"


. numlist "3.878"

. display "`r(numlist)'"
3.878
```

You will remember from above that the best way of entering a single number is in a scalar. We will cover scalars later in the session.

However, when you enter two or more numbers, display doesn't work very well. The numberlist is correctly stored, but it will not display properly using this syntax which worked for a single number.

```
numlist "3.878 8.8797"
display "`r(numlist)'"

. numlist "3.878 8.8797"

.
. display "`r(numlist)'"
3.878 8.8797
```

You have to use a loop to display a numberlist if it contains more than one element.

Loops are covered in detail later in the course. For the moment, you will just need to understand the basic architecture of a loop. Unfortunately, loops and macros are often used together (as in this example). The loop begins with an instruction to Stata to examine each element of the list of numbers you have put into the macro called numlist. The end of that line begins with an open curly bracket. The next line tells Stata what operation to perform on the item that has been retrieved in the previous line. The whole loop is closed with a closed curly bracket on a line by itself.

```
numlist "3.878 8.8797"
foreach i in `r(numlist)' {
        display "`i'"
        }


. numlist "3.878 8.8797"

. foreach i in `r(numlist)' {
  2.       display "`i'"
  3.       }
3.878
8.8797
```

You can enter lists or series of numbers.

```
numlist "1(2)10"

foreach i in `r(numlist)'{
display "`i'"
}


. foreach i in `r(numlist)'{
  2. display "`i'"
  3. }
1
3
5
7
9
```

You can use a disjointed list, or enter numbers individually

```
numlist "1/5 25 8.8873"

foreach i in `r(numlist)'{
display "`i'"
}

. numlist "1/5 25 8.8873"

.
. foreach i in `r(numlist)'{
  2. display "`i'"
  3. }
1
2
3
4
5
25
8.88735
```

To see your numberlist, use:

```
return list

return list
macros:
                              r(numlist) : "1 2 3 4 5 25 8.8873"
```

It is not possible to delete the numlist manually. It will disappear once you exit Stata. It is of little importance, however, if you always define your new numlist before you use it, then there's very little chance of you mixing up your lists.

You can create the list and loop simultaneously. If you have a series of numbers, then forvalues will work as below.

```
forvalues i = 1(2)10{
display " `I' "
}

. forvalues i = 1(2)10{
  2.       display "`i' "
  3.       }
1
3
5
7
9
```

If you have a set of individual unconnected numbers, then foreach is the loop to use.

```
foreach i in 1 10 2993 83942.839427{
display "`i'"
}


. foreach i in 1 10 2993 83942.839427{
  2. display "`i'"
  3. }
1
10
2993
83942.839427
```

NOTE: The transient numberlist in a foreach loop disappears at the end of the loop, so you don't have to worry about their management and/or deletion separately.

b. Scalars

We have previously encountered scalars. The expression may hold either a numeric or a string expression. Scalars can hold reasonably long strings, even longer than those held in macros, and unlike macros, can also hold binary data. We will cover the use of scalars for numeric data in this section and that for strings later on. This is because the syntax involved is different.

To enter a number into a scalar, use the following straightforward syntax. I will give the scalar an arbitrary name of length as you can assume that I wish to enter a single number into the scalar that represents a length that I will need later on in my analysis. For this example, I am using the length of the Severn Bridge in metres.

```
tempname length
scalar `length' = 1600
scalar list
display 3*`length'
display 2+`length'

 . tempname length

 . scalar `length' = 1600

 . scalar list
     000000 =   1600

 . display 3*`length'
4800

 . display 2+`length'
 1602
```

Now that the program has run, scalar has disappeared. This is a foolproof way of ensuring that your temporary entities are not lingering around the programming environment.

c. Local Macros

A local macro is present for as long as the program creating it is being run, but then it disappears. So, you may wonder, why go to all the trouble of creating a tempvar and then a scalar to accomplish this? Macros are not good at holding numbers for a complicated number of reasons. However, there is at least one occasion in which you do need a macro to hold a number, and that is when you are putting a temporary number into a filepath. We are covering the syntax of entering numbers into filepaths next. For the moment, it's very important to learn the syntax of macros.

Be aware that you cannot combine tempvar with macros. This is not so much of an issue with local macros as the macro disappears once the program is run, so you have to make sure that you use different names for macros within each program, or the subsequent local macros will overwrite the preceding ones without giving any alert.

Global macros persist, and this is where the real danger lies. If you define a global macro in one program and completely forget about it, you can easily overwrite its contents without realising it in a subsequent program. Great caution is therefore warranted when using global macros. We are reviewing global macros later, so we will revisit this issue then. However, this is the main reason why you list all your global macros in one convenient place (usually at the top of the Master file).

The syntax begins with the type of macro you are going to use. In this case, we tell Stata that we want a local macro, that its name is going to be "year" and that it is going to hold the number 2019.

Once we create the macro and the script is run, the macro disappears. So we often check that the macro is holding the correct variable by displaying its contents immediately after its creation.

If you have entered a single number, to display it you need to place ' and ' before and after the local macro name. The names for these symbols are "backtick" and "apostrophe", respectively.

```
local year 2019
display `year'


. local year 2019

. display `year'
2019
```

An alternative syntax which some people prefer because it indicates that you are entering a number is to use an equal sign. However, it works only when you are entering one number, and once you start to enter two or more, Stata will throw an error. For this reason, I prefer not to use this syntax. Equal signs are used in macros, and we will encounter them later when we running an operation within a macro. But more on that anon. To avoid confusion, I would recommend you **DO NOT** use equal signs to enter these types of data into macros. We will encounter equal signs with macros later, and in these instances, you will discover that Stata evaluates the contents of the macro and what you get out can depend on what's inside the macro. We will deal with this later, but if what you want to get out is exactly what you put into a macro, then do not use equal signs.

Enter several numbers and see how the macro operates.

```
local years 2019 2020
display `years' 20192020

foreach i of local years{
display `i'
}

. local years 2019 2020

. display `years'
20192020

.
. foreach i of local years{
  2. display `i'
  3. }
2019
2020
```

The output from the first display command is not satisfactory as the output has run the two years together. The second command using a display within a loop has correctly separated and displayed the two numbers sequentially. This often causes problems because you don't want to go to the trouble of writing a loop every time you want to display its contents. This is where the importance of displaying macros comes into its own. The issue you have to overcome is that the macro contains a space that you want Stata to display. To display the contents of this macro correctly, you need to use the following syntax. This is where the display syntax for macros gets tricky.

To include the space in your display, you have to tell Stata that the macro contains a space. This is done by activating the formatting built in within Stat's display command. In this case we start and close with quotation marks and put the backtick and apostrophe inside them. When Stata reads this, it starts with the outside symbols in pairs and then reads inwards. It reads the quotation marks as indicating that spaces within the macro should be reproduced in the display. Then it reads the backtick and the apostrophe to tell it that it's dealing with a **local** macro (and not a variable or a global macro, for example).

```
local years 2019 2020
display "`years´"



. local years 2019 2020

. display "`years'"
2019 2020
```

Sometimes, when you receive data that needs to be processed in your analysis, the variable names and/or file names come enclosed in quotation marks.

Infuriatingly, Stata sometimes puts the file names into quotation marks itself without any prompting, so you have to learn to deal with this scenario as well. Let's assume you have two numbers that have been enclosed within quotation marks that you wish to place into a macro named years. The objects are the years "2019" and "2020". This requires more attention because the display command will interpret the quotation marks as special characters, and it will not produce the correct results. In this case, we need to alert Stata to the fact that quotation marks are included and that it should reproduce these (as well as the space and treating the contents as a local macro and not a variable name). Phew.

In fact, this syntax works remarkably well for displaying all local macros (containing numbers as well as strings). Stata doesn't care if you warn it that the macro contains special characters and/or a space, and then it finds that no such special characters and/or spaces exist. The solution is therefore to use this complicated syntax whenever you can, as it's likely the only one you will have to learn for the majority of situations. With at least one exception. When you are using macros in filepaths, the display changes a bit, and we will discuss this later. But for the moment, if you learn this syntax for displaying local macros, then you can't go far wrong. To put the items (for example the years 2019 and 2020) into the local macro we begin with quotation marks to tell Stata this is where we are starting the macro. In fact, you can use quotation marks whenever you enter data into most types of macros (and we will use them all the time when we are entering string variables). However, they are not used when we enter variable names that are already created in a dataset. Don't worry about this complication for the moment. We will cover this later.

```
local years `" "2019" "2020" "'
display `"`years'"'


. local years `" "2019" "2020" "'

. display `"`years'"'
 "2019" "2020"
```

Notice that you can leave a space between the quotation marks and the years when you input the data into the local, but you *cannot* leave any spaces between the punctuation marks and the name of the macro when you are displaying its contents. It's better not to leave any spaces at all between the punctuation marks and the contents either when you are displaying or when you are entering data into macros.

d. Global Macros

Now we move on to global macros, which will be much easier now you've got an understanding of how to handle local macros. Entering data into global macros is identical to that for local macros except you define the macro with the prefix global. Displaying the data is very similar. You use the same syntax of "' '" before and after the macro to display it, but you also need to tell Stata that this is a global macro. This is done by placing the symbols ${ before the macro and the symbol } afterwards. The syntax with the local macro is very similar. You use the same outer two characters before and after the display command. The inner ' and ' (which tell Stata that the contents are a local macro) are removed and replaced with symbols that tell Stata that it is dealing with a global macro.

```
global year 2019
display `"${year}"'

global years 2019 2020
display `"${years}"'

global years `" "2019" "2020" "'
display `"${years}"'

. global year 2019
. display `"${year}"'
2019

. global years 2019 2020
. display `"${years}"'
2019 2020

. global years `" "2019" "2020" "'
. display `"${years}"'
"2019" "2020"
```

You have had to use seven punctuation symbols to display this macro correctly, and this is a huge stumbling block to the correct use of macros and a reason why some programmers do not use them routinely. They are complicated, and they require a significant amount of patience, but you will be well rewarded. A program written with macros and displayed correctly displays a level of familiarity with Stata that reassures a reviewer of your code, makes the code more efficient and is much easier to read.

e. Entering Macros Containing Numbers into Filepaths

Let's create a macro containing a single number and try to put this into a filepath. In reality, you are much more likely to try to create a numberlist and put those successively into a filepath if you have folders that differ from each other by a number in their name; for example, "01_ECG", "02_ECG" ... .. "12_ECG". You will need to loop through these numbers and enter the number component of the filepath as a macro.

Let's start with a simple example: create a macro with a number and display the contents of the macro as you would to ensure that the macro is holding what you would expect it to. I always display my macros after creating them to check.

```
local number 3
display `"`number'"'


. local number 3

. display `"`number'"'
3
```

Now, let's try to enter this number into a filepath and display the filepath.

```
local number 3
display "C:\somefolder\somefolder\`number'_ECG\somefile.dta"


. display "C:\somefolder\somefolder\`number'_ECG\somefile.dta"
C:\somefolder\somefolder`number'_ECG\somefile.dta
```

Notice that I have used **backslash** as the separator because this is the default used by the Windows system and the style that you are likely to copy and paste to your directory of interest. The issue is that the backslash character when placed before a macro instructs Stata to skip over the macro. This is considered useful in some very high-level programming, but we are not considering these instances in this book. If you are particularly interested, the Stata manual gives some excellent examples, but they are not for the faint-hearted.

There are two solutions. The one I favour is to manually change all the hyphens from backslash to forward slash. That way you are consistent in your programming when you start to use R. The second method is to precede the offending hyphen with yet another backslash (i.e. to use double backslash before a macro). Both exemplars are given below.

```
local number 3
display "C:/somefolder/somefolder/`number'_ECG/somefile.dta"
display "C:\somefolder\somefolder\\`number'_ECG\somefile.dta"


. display "C:/somefolder/somefolder/`number'_ECG/somefile.dta"
C:/somefolder/somefolder/3_ECG/somefile.dta

. display "C:\somefolder\somefolder\\`number'_ECG\somefile.dta"
C:\somefolder\somefolder\3_ECG\somefile.dta
```

III. DEALING WITH STORAGE OF VARIABLES AND STRINGS

a. Local Macros

Let's enter the following series of words into the local macro called objects – telephone, lamp, calculator and computer.

```
local objects `" telephone lamp calculator computer "'
display `"`objects'"'


. local objects `" telephone lamp calculator computer "'

. display `"`objects'"'
telephone lamp calculator computer
```

Now, let's enter these words surrounded by quotation marks into a macro. This is important as the file names you will need to manipulate when you analyse electronic health records frequently come enclosed in quotation marks, and it's critical that you're comfortable with handling them. When you are manipulating variables in a dataset, you will not wish to have the quotation marks. You will just treat the variable names as you usually would. However, if the macros are being used to read names of files that you are manipulating, the quotation marks are necessary, as once Stata reads files, it will add quotation marks, but not so if it's reading variables. This will be explained later once we start to do some practice exercises.

```
local objects `" "telephone" "lamp" "calculator" "computer" "'
di `"`objects'"'


. local objects `" "telephone" "lamp" "calculator" "computer" "'

. di `"`objects'"'
"telephone" "lamp" "calculator" "computer"
```

To enter variables into a macro, you do not use any quotation marks.

```
clear
sysuse auto
local variables rep78 price
foreach i of local variables{
summ `i'
}
clear


clear

. sysuse auto
(1978 Automobile Data)

. local variables rep78 price

. foreach i of local variables{
 2. summ `i'
 3. }

    Variable |       Obs        Mean    Std. Dev.       Min        Max
-------------+--------------------------------------------------------
       rep78 |        69    3.405797    .9899323          1          5

    Variable |       Obs        Mean    Std. Dev.       Min        Max
-------------+--------------------------------------------------------
       price |        74    6165.257    2949.496       3291      15906
. clear
```

b. Global Macros

Let's create a global macro holding the objects listed above and display the contents.

```
global objects `" "telephone" "lamp" "calculator" "computer" "'
display `"${objects}"'
macro drop _all

. global objects `" "telephone" "lamp" "calculator" "computer" "'

. display `"${objects}"'
 "telephone" "lamp" "calculator" "computer"

. macro drop _all
```

It is a good idea to always drop your global macros once you have used them if you don't require them later.

To hold variable names in a global macro:

```
clear
sysuse auto
global variables rep78 price
display `"${variables}"' rep78 price
clear
macro drop _all


. clear

. sysuse auto
(1978 Automobile Data)

. global variables rep78 price

. display `"${variables}"'
rep78 price

. clear
```

c. Scalars

Scalars are not normally used to hold text. It's much better to place variable names and text into a macro. I demonstrate here how to use scalars in this way, but I would not recommend this usage. As usual, I take the precaution of using a tempname to ensure I'm not accidentally over writing a previously declared scalar.

```
tempname object
scalar `object' = "Telephone"
display `object'


. tempname object

. scalar `object' = "Telephone"

. display `object'
Telephone
```

d. Entering Macros Containing Strings into Filepaths

Let's try to enter a local macro into a filepath.

```
local prefix `"a"'
display `"`prefix'"'
display "local_data/`prefix'_dataset/files"
display "local_data\`prefix'_dataset/files"
display "local_data\\`prefix'_dataset/files"


. local prefix `"a"'
. display `"`prefix'"'
a
. display "local_data/`prefix'_dataset/files"
local_data/a_dataset/files

. display "local_data\`prefix'_dataset/files"
local_data`prefix'_dataset/files

. display "local_data\\`prefix'_dataset/files"
local_data\a_dataset/files
```

Note that when displaying a macro that is inside a filepath, you strip off the double quotes. This rule applies to both local and global macros.

You will note that it is much easier to manipulate forward slashes than backslashes when using local macros. If you insist on using backslashes, then you must use a double backslash where it occurs just before a macro (global or local).

Now let's have a look at inserting global macros into filepaths.

Just a reminder that global macros are more enduring than local macros in Stata's memory and are transferred in memory across environments. The work environment has a special meaning in computer science and will take on great importance if you program in R. For Stata users, it's not so important, so we will not spend any more time on it. Just be aware that global macros can be overwritten accidentally by later contents, and you should be exceedingly careful with them.

```
global prefix    `"a"'
display `"${prefix}"'
display  "local_data/${prefix}_dataset/files"
display  "local_data\${prefix}_dataset\files"
display "local_data\\${prefix}_dataset/files"
macro drop _all

. global prefix `"a"'

. display `"${prefix}"'
a

. display "local_data/${prefix}_dataset/files"
local_data/a_dataset/files

. display "local_data\${prefix}_dataset\files"
local_data${prefix}_dataset\files

. display "local_data\\${prefix}_dataset/files"
local_data\a_dataset/files

. macro drop _all
```

Recall that you need a double backslash before a macro, or Stata will think the single backslash is an escape character and will ignore it. Also note that since I have created a global macro, I take care to drop it when I no longer need it.

IV. EXTENDED MACRO FUNCTIONS

As if local and global macros are not confusing enough, you can expand their functionality. This is essential when you are using electronic health records. For the moment, although it may appear tiresome, I will review some of the many extended functions that are available for Stata. For more information and complete list, you can use Stata's inbuilt help function. I will demonstrate the most commonly used functions.

Change your directory to the root folder of the course (for example, if you have exited Stata since you last changed your working directory) and check that your present working directory (pwd) is correct.

```
cd "C:/Analysis_Folder"
pwd


. cd "C:/Analysis_Folder"
C:\Analysis_Folder

. pwd C:\Analysis_Folder
```

These extended functions work very similarly for both local and global macros, so I will demonstrate their use only in local macros. It is a good habit to not use global macros unless only absolutely necessary and very sparingly at that. They pollute your environment unless you are very careful.

The following extended functions are commonly encountered. There are several others that are not so commonly encountered in analyses of electronic health records. If you are particularly interested in these, then type "help macro" into the Stata window and then click on the hyperlink for the associated .pdf file.

One of the key operations that needs to be mastered very early on is how to find files in a folder on your computer and then import them into Stata. This task is broken down into locating the files and importing their names into Stata. The next section on loops will show you how to use the names of the files you have stored in your macro to import the files, put them into temporary storage and append them. **Append** is the term Stata uses to add more observations to a dataset. When you are adding more variables to an existing dataset from another dataset, the term used in Stata is **"merge"**.

a. Obtaining Lists of Files in a Folder

Assume that the folder named "01_Data_In" contains a folder entitled "Station_Data" and "Data_Download_1" is contained within this folder. .csv and .txt and very commonly encountered data types. Assume that the folder "Data_Download_1" contains a folder named "Excel", which contains files that we will eventually import and append together to get one dataset for later analysis.

```
local input_files: dir "`c(pwd)'/Data_In/Station_Data/Data_Download_1/Excel"
files"*", /// respectcase
display `"`input_files'"'

. local input_files: dir "`c(pwd)'/Data_In/Station_Data/Data_Download_1/Excel"
> files "*", ///
> respectcase

. display `"`input_files'"'
"A0YT4H.csv" "A2HW6A.csv" "A3EK7O.csv" "A3JW3X.csv" "A4DR3B.csv" "A4DS4Y.csv" "A4KO8Q.csv"
"A4ZU5N.csv" "A5ND5O.csv" "A5RZ8J.csv" "A5ZB9C.csv" "A6YU2I.csv" "A7CX3P.csv" "A8AE0E.csv"
"A8KR0M.csv" "B0AE9X.csv" "B1JW5F.csv" "B1QX1J.csv" "B1WN3Q.csv" "B3AI4H.csv" "B5QZ5T.csv"
"B6LQ1C.csv" "B6OS3D.csv" "B6UJ0A.csv" "B6ZN1J.csv" "B7CD9F.csv" "B8XW1A.csv" "C1IN8C.csv"
"C1PH5U.csv" "C2DJ8U.csv" "C3SF2A.csv" "C4PI7U.................................................................
```

Note that I have used the syntax of 'c(pwd)' in front of the filepath to give a dynamic relative filepath. Strictly speaking this isn't absolutely necessary as Stata already knows what your working directory is, so you could have inputted a relative filepath (relative to your working directory) by omitting the 'c(pwd)'. Having said this, putting in the full path is a good habit as sometimes Stata will not understand where to save the files when we start looping without a complete filepath. The file name invokes the wildcard * to include all files. If you wanted all files beginning with the letter A, you would use "A*", for example.

You should also note the option of "respectcase" is invoked. Unless you do so, Stata will convert all the characters it encounters to lowercase. It's not really important in this case, but if you are converting .csv files to .dta, it makes sense to have the resultant output files identically named.

b. Using Stata's Inbuilt String Manipulation Functions

Now that you have the list of files in memory, you may want to convert them to .dta files for easier manipulation. However, Stata has the suffix ".csv" already in its memory, so your resultant files could easily be named "Example.csv.dta". It's necessary to manipulate the names stored in your macro so as to remove the .csv extension. Stata's extended string functions for macros will accomplish this for you.

Once again store the file names in the Windows directory into a local macro and then create another macro with the names that have had their extension stripped off.

```
local input_files: dir "`c(pwd)'/Data_In/Station_Data/Data_Download_1/Excel" files "*",
respectcase
local output_files: subinstr local input_files ".csv" "", all
display `"`output_files'"'


local output_files: subinstr local input_files ".csv" "", all

. display `"`output_files'"'
"A0YT4H" "A2HW6A" "A3EK7O" "A3JW3X" "A4DR3B" "A4DS4Y" "A4KO8Q" "A4ZU5N" "A5ND5O" "A5RZ8J"
"A5ZB9C" "A6YU2I" "A7CX3P" "A8AE0E" "A8KR0M" "B0AE9X" "B1JW5F" "B1QX1J" "B1WN3Q" "B3AI4H"
"B5QZ5T" "B6LQ1C" "B6OS3D" "B6UJ0A" "B6ZN1J" "B7CD9F" "B8XW1A" "C1IN8C" "C1PH5U" "C2DJ8U"
"C3SF2A" "C4PI7U" "C4WP9U" "C4WV8G" "C5JZ0V" "C5VJ3H" "C6WN3W" "C7QZ1D" "C7WA5G" "C8LV9A"
"C9PP9K" "D0MS2Y" "D1B J5J" "D1QR8L" "D2ND3Q" "D3KF9G" "D4JU5E" "D5XP9T
```

Note the use of the option "all". This tells Stata to perform the operation on all files in the local macro.

c. Counting

You will need to know how many files are in the folder so that you can tell Stata how many to import when you come to writing your loop. You could easily open the folder in Windows and count them (or the count of the files is also displayed in the bottom left-hand side of the window in the Windows OS). You could possibly enter this number into your loop. Often the number of files will change, for example, with the addition of more data. If you enter the number itself of the count into the loop, Stata will ignore the files that are listed after this number.

If you happen to have removed any files, Stata will report an error as it will not be able to find the missing files. Entering a fixed number into a loop is an example of hardcoding, which is poor programming practice. If, however, you use Stata's extended function to count the number of files and then to import them using this number, you can vary the number of files in a folder effortlessly. In this example, the code already used above is extended so as to create another local macro named "count", which will hold the count of the number of files in the folder.

```
local input_files: dir "`c(pwd)'/Data_In/Station_Data/Data_Download_1/Excel" files
"*", respectcase
local output_files: subinstr local input_files ".csv" "", all
local count: word count `output_files'
display `"`count'"'



. local input_files: dir "`c(pwd)'/Data_In/Station_Data/Data_Download_1/Excel"
> files "*", respectcase

. local output_files: subinstr local input_files ".csv" "", all

. local count: word count `output_files'

. display `"`count'"'
333
```

The command subinstr is Stata contraction for "substitute in string". The first input is the string you wish to consider (viz. the contents of the local name "input_files"). The second input is the sequence of characters you wish Stata to identify (".csv"). The third input "" signifies that you wish to replace it with nothing at all.

If you wished simply to display the identified characters you would use the command "substr" which we will shortly encounter.

d. Labels

Obtaining labels for variables and values can be frustrating in Stata. It's easier to use macros when extracting and storing this information.

Let's extract the label for a variable using the inbuilt auto dataset.

```
sysuse auto
local rep78_label: variable label rep78
display `"`rep78_label'"'


. sysuse auto
(1978 Automobile Data)

. local rep78_label: variable label rep78

. display `"`rep78_label'"'
Repair Record 1978
```

The variable "foreign" is a categorical label. It therefore has both value names as well as a label name. The label name is the name of the entity that contains the values. The label names are the names associated with the values for the variable. This is slightly confusing, but it's well worth the effort to understand this by looking at Stata's help files.

To display the levels of the variable, use the following syntax.

```
local foreign_value_label: value label foreign
display `"`foreign_value_label'"'


. local foreign_value_label: value label foreign

. display `"`foreign_value_label'"'
origin
```

Specifying the option missing ensures that levels of values with no values are returned. However, these levels have labels that you may wish to use as well.

```
levelsof foreign, local(foreign_levels) missing
foreach i of local foreign_levels{
local label: label origin `i'
display `"`label'"'
}
clear

. levels of foreign, local(foreign_levels) missing
0 1

. foreach i of local foreign_levels{
 2. local label: label origin `i'
 3. display `"`label'"'
 4.      }
Domestic
Foreign
```

Note: First the value labels are put into a local macro, and then the contents of this macro are displayed within a loop. It is possible to display the value labels without going to the trouble of putting them into a macro first, and this is covered in the section entitled "Advanced Macros".

The dataset sometimes carries a label, and you can access this.

```
sysuse auto2
local data_label: data label
display `"`data_label'"'
clear

. sysuse auto2
(1978 Automobile Data)

. local data_label: data label

. display `"`data_label'"'
1978 Automobile Data
```

V. ADVANCED MACRO FUNCTIONS

a. Putting One Macro into Another

It is possible to insert macros into other macros (but why you would want to do this is unclear). However, for reasons of completeness, I describe this process here:

```
local number 5
local number2        `number'
display `"`number2'"'

. local number 5

. local number2`number'

. display `"`number2'"'
5
```

You can make up commands and run them as a macro if you use that command often (e.g. options).

NOTE: Since you are using the macro as a command, there are NO inner quotation marks.

```
local drop `" drop if type ==1 "'
sysuse sandstone.dta, clear
codebook type

`drop'

codebook type
clear


. local drop `" drop if type ==1 "'

. sysuse sandstone.dta, clear
(Subsea elevation of Lamont sandstone in an area of Ohio)

. codebook type

--------------------------------------------------------------------
type                                  Type of collection methods
--------------------------------------------------------------------

           type: numeric (byte)
          label: collection

          range: [1,3]                     units: 1
  unique values: 3                     missing .: 0/6,400

     tabulation: Freq.   Numeric  Label
                    17         1  measured
                    59         2  estimated
                 6,324         3  interpolated

.
. `drop'
(17 observations deleted)

.
. codebook type

--------------------------------------------------------------------
type                                  Type of collection methods
--------------------------------------------------------------------

           type: numeric (byte)
          label: collection

          range: [2,3]                     units: 1
  unique values: 2                     missing .: 0/6,383

     tabulation: Freq.   Numeric  Label
                    59         2  estimated
                 6,324         3  interpolated

. clear
```

b. How to Evaluate an Expression and Place the Results into a Macro

In this example, we will use the auto dataset again. You can download this dataset by using the command "webuse auto, clear" First, we will display the contents of an evaluated macro (without keeping the macro). Then we will alter the contents of an evaluated macro (again without retaining the macro) in one step. Since we are using an extended function, the syntax includes the full colon (:). If we were evaluating an expression, we would use the equal sign.

Here we will display the variable label associated with the variable "make".

```
sysuse auto, clear
display "`:variable label make'"


. sysuse auto, clear
(1978 Automobile Data)

. display "`:variable label make'"
Make and Model
```

Now, we will display the first four letters of the first word in the variable label for the variable "make".

```
displaysubstr ("`:variable label make'", 1,4 )


. display substr("`:variable label make'", 1,4 )
Make
```

This is the same procedure in two steps.

```
local name = substr("`:variable label make'", 1,4)
display `"`name'"'


. local name = substr("`:variable label make'", 1,4)

. display `"`name'"'
Make
```

NOTE: You have the evaluation of a macro within a display within a local macro. This is quite complicated programming. Also note that you have used an equal sign as substr is not an extended macro function (therefore you cannot use a full colon).

c. A Salutary Example of Paying Attention to Equal Signs

```
local word `"upper(frog)"'
display `"`word'"'

local word `= upper("frog")'
display `"`word'"'


. local word `"upper(frog)"'

. display `"`word'"'
upper(frog)

.
. local word `= upper("frog")'

. display `"`word'"'
FROG
```

Tokenize divides a string into tokens, storing the result in 1',2', ... (the positional local macros). So you can refer to the strings as numbers. This makes it easy to parse a list of words. This feature is rarely used in the analysis of electronic health records and is included here for completeness.

```
tokenize apple computer
display `" `1´ `2´ "´ apple computer

tokenize `" "Stata good" "R bad" "'
display `" "`1'" "`2'" "'

tokenize "Grade A++"
display `" "`1'" "`2'" "`3'" "'


tokenize "Grade A++", parse ("+")
display `" "`1'" "`2'" "`3'" "'

        while "`*'" != ""{

        display `" "`*'" "'
        macro shift
        }

.
. tokenize apple computer

. display `" `1´ `2´ "´ apple computer
`1´ `2´ "´ apple computer

. tokenize `" "Stata good" "R bad" "'

. display `" "`1'" "`2'" "'
"Stata good" "R bad"

. tokenize "Grade A++"

. display `" "`1'" "`2'" "`3'" "'
"Grade" "A++" ""

. tokenize "Grade A++", parse ("+")

. display `" "`1'" "`2'" "`3'" "'
"Grade A" "+" "+"

.
.       while "`*'" != ""{
 2.
.       display `" "`*'" "'
 3.       macro shift
 4.       }
"Grade A + +"
"+ +"
"+"
```

VI. RETURN LISTS

a. creturn List

This is a bit complicated. Sometimes Stata stores variables as numbers and sometimes as strings. It's not easy to figure out what you are dealing with, but it is important to know the difference as it affects the way you can manipulate them. Stata has a value stored for pi. As you would imagine, this is stored and manipulated as a number. Stata has a value stored for the alphabet. This is stored as a string. There is also a value stored for time. Let's have a look at some examples that may clarify. Confusingly although these values persist in Stata's memory, they are called and manipulated as though they are LOCAL macros and NOT global macros.

To display the current time:

```
display `"`c(current_time)'"'


. display `"`c(current_time)'"'
16:34:23
```

To display a greeting with the current time:

```
if c(current_time) < "12:00:00" {
local greeting "Good Morning"
}

else if c(current_time) >= "12:00:00" & c(current_time) < "17:00:00" {
local greeting "Good Afternoon"
}

else if c(current_time) >= "17:00:00" & c(current_time) < "19:00:00" {
local greeting "Good Evening"
}

else{
local greeting "Good Night Irene"
}

display `"`greeting'"'


. if c(current_time) < "12:00:00" {
. local greeting "Good Morning"
. }
.
. else if c(current_time) >= "12:00:00" & c(current_time) < "17:00:00" {
. local greeting "Good Afternoon"
. }

.
. else if c(current_time) >= "17:00:00" & c(current_time) < "19:00:00"{
. local greeting "Good Evening"
. }

.
. else{
. local greeting "Good Night Irene"
. }
.
.
. display `"`greeting'"'
Good Afternoon
```

b. eretun Lists

This type of return lists the results of **estimation** commands such as regress and logistic. On average, you can think of them as being the elements that are estimated when you fit statistical models. These elements are present in memory until they are displaced by the next model (not necessarily the next Stata command). These results are often accessed and displayed. The issues with displaying these results are discussed later in this course.

c. return lists

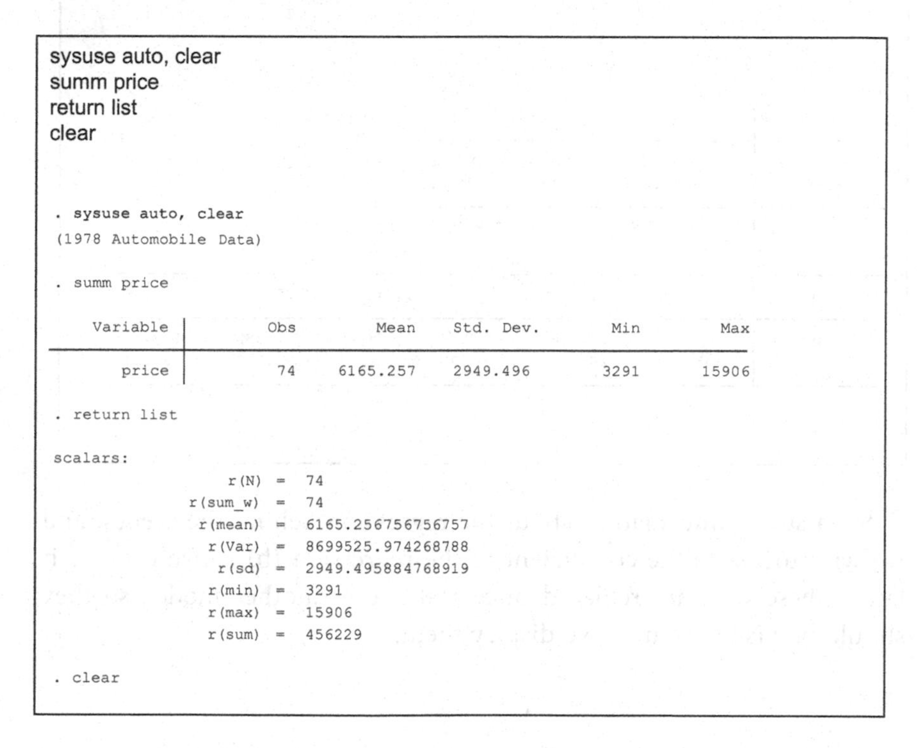

```
sysuse auto, clear
summm price
return list
clear
```

```
. sysuse auto, clear
(1978 Automobile Data)

. summm price

    Variable |        Obs        Mean    Std. Dev.       Min        Max
-------------+---------------------------------------------------------
       price |         74    6165.257    2949.496       3291      15906

. return list

scalars:
                  r(N) =  74
              r(sum_w) =  74
               r(mean) =  6165.256756756757
                r(Var) =  8699525.974268788
                 r(sd) =  2949.495884768919
                r(min) =  3291
                r(max) =  15906
                r(sum) =  456229

. clear
```

You have encountered return lists when we reviewed the creation and deletion of numberlists. You can also display saved results with this command.

d. sreturn Lists

This entity holds programming information, and you can use it if you wish to record the specifics of the computing environment in which your code was executed. It is very rarely used. Use the command "macro list".

VII. MATRICES

Some results come in the form of matrices, and it's necessary to be able to manipulate them. Let's see how the price of a car varies with its length using the dataset auto2.

```
sysuse auto
regress price length

. sysuse auto
(1978 Automobile Data)

. regress price   length

      Source |       SS           df       MS      Number of obs   =        74
-------------+----------------------------------   F(1, 72)        =     16.50
       Model |  118425867         1   118425867   Prob > F        =    0.0001
    Residual |  516639529        72  7175549.01   R-squared       =    0.1865
-------------+----------------------------------   Adj R-squared   =    0.1752
       Total |  635065396        73  8699525.97   Root MSE        =    2678.7

------------------------------------------------------------------------------
       price |      Coef.   Std. Err.      t    P>|t|     [95% Conf. Interval]
-------------+----------------------------------------------------------------
      length |   57.20224   14.08047     4.06   0.000     29.13332    85.27115
       _cons |  -4584.899   2664.437    -1.72   0.090    -9896.357     726.559
------------------------------------------------------------------------------
```

Stata stores information about the regression behind the scenes, and we wish to locate the co-efficient of the regression (b) so we can use it later. These data are replaced once Stata runs another model, so they should be visible to us if we display them.

ereturn list

```
. ereturn list

scalars:
                  e(N) =  74
               e(df_m) =  1
               e(df_r) =  72
                  e(F) =  16.5040845075474
                 e(r2) =  .1864782241337118
               e(rmse) =  2678.721525601992
                e(mss) =  118425867.2775322
                e(rss) =  516639528.8440893
               e(r2_a) =  .1751793105800135
                 e(ll) =  -688.0767132700388
               e(ll_0) =  -695.7128688987767
               e(rank) =  2

macros:
            e(cmdline) : "regress price length"
              e(title) : "Linear regression"
          e(marginsok) : "XB default"
                e(vce) : "ols"
             e(depvar) : "price"
                e(cmd) : "regress"
         e(properties) : "b V"
            e(predict) : "regres_p"
              e(model) : "ols"
          e(estat_cmd) : "regress_estat"

matrices:
                  e(b) :  1 x 2
                  e(V) :  2 x 2

functions:
             e(sample)
```

Observe that towards the bottom of the printout, Stata has displayed that it has two matrices in memory: that of the coefficients and that of the variance matrix. We're interested in the first of the two coefficients ([1,1] in matrix notation).

To display the matrices:

Matrix list e(b)

```
. matrix list e(b)

e(b)[1,2]
        length       _cons
y1   57.202238   -4584.899
```

Observe that unlike local macros and return lists, ereturn list does not exit memory until you run another **estimation** command.

Most people are more concerned with the list of coefficients. You often need to report these values. We will review how to extract these elements here, and the next section will discuss how to display them.

Looking back at the matrix of coefficients, you will observe that these are named by Stata. To extract the coefficients, you will need to use the names assigned by Stata and place them into scalars before you display them.

```
tempname length_coefficient
scalar `length_coefficient' = _b[length]
display `length_coefficient'

. tempname length_coefficient

. scalar `length_coefficient' = _b[length]
. display `length_coefficient'
57.202238
```

If you need to use the scalar much later in your analysis, then omit the step of creating a temporary name or the entity will disappear once the program is run. I would recommend making a list of scalars at the top of your master program file (where you have your list of global macros) so as to keep a note of them and ensure you are not overwriting a value accidentally by naming two entities identically.

While the matrices that are returned by ereturn do give the coefficients, the p values and standard errors of the estimation often need to be reported. For this reason, I would suggest you not use ereturn postestimation.

Not only does Stata hold values that are accessed by the postestimation command of ereturn list. You will also find that Stata holds values in another class of temporary storage, which you can view by issuing the return list command.

Stata has very helpfully created a table in memory of the most useful values you are likely to need. Not so helpfully, the commands to extract it are not commonly known and less well documented. The values are stored in a matrix, which is named as a table, which is retained until another estimation command is used. To display the table: The first thing to do is to store the contents of the table into a matrix.

```
matrix table = r(table)
matrix list table

. matrix table = r(table)

. matrix list table

table[9,2]
            length       _cons
     b   57.202238   -4584.899
    se   14.080475    2664.437
     t   4.0625219  -1.7207759
pvalue    .0001222   .08958651
    ll   29.133325   -9896.357
    ul   85.271152     726.559
    df          72          72
```

Again, it's relatively straightforward to identify and store the elements of the table that you need. In this case, let's remove the coefficient and standard error for length from the matrix and store these in two scalars. Matrices are indexed by two numbers in square brackets separated by a comma. The first number indicates the row number, and the second indicates the column number.

```
tempname length_b
tempname length_se
scalar `length_b' = table[1,1]
display `length_b'
scalar `length_se' = table[2,1]
display `length_se'


. tempname length_b

. tempname length_se

. scalar `length_b' = table[1,1]

. display `length_b'
57.202238

. scalar `length_se' = table[2,1]

. display `length_se'
14.080475
```

Remember that the matrix you have created is still present, and you will need to delete it manually.

```
matrix drop table
```

VIII. DISPLAYING AND FORMATTING RESULTS

You have now learnt how to extract items from Stata's postestimation variables. Now, we will cover how to display them. You will need to display the results you have obtained appropriately. The postestimation results are often stored with too many decimal places. You need to **format** the results. The % sign indicates to Stata that you are formatting the number that follows. To get two decimal places and three decimal places, respectively, follow the syntax below. It is intuitive, and you usually only ever use a limited number of formats. A simple rule of thumb is to determine the number of decimal places that you want first. That number goes after the full stop in the formatting command. Add one to the number you have decided on for the number of decimal places, and then add again the number of places before the decimal place. So to show a number with two numbers before and three numbers after the decimal place, I would use %6.3fc (f means fixed formatting and c means use a comma if appropriate).

Note the words are embedded within multiple sets of quotation marks, and the scalars are formatted immediately preceding each number.

```
clear
sysuse auto
regress price length
matrix table = r(table)
tempname length_b
tempname length_se
scalar `length_b' = table[1,1]
display `length_b' 57.202238
scalar     `length_se' = table[2,1]
display `length_b'
display "The coefficient of length in the regression is " `length_b' "."
display "The coefficient of length in the regression is " %3.2f `length_b' "
display "The standard error is " %3.2f `length_se' "."
matrix drop _all
clear
```

```
. clear

. sysuse auto
(1978 Automobile Data)

. regress price length

      Source |       SS           df       MS      Number of obs   =        74
-------------+----------------------------------   F(1, 72)        =     16.50
       Model |   118425867         1   118425867   Prob > F        =    0.0001
    Residual |   516639529        72  7175549.01   R-squared       =    0.1865
-------------+----------------------------------   Adj R-squared   =    0.1752
       Total |   635065396        73  8699525.97   Root MSE        =    2678.7

------------------------------------------------------------------------------
       price |      Coef.   Std. Err.      t    P>|t|     [95%Conf.  Interval]
-------------+----------------------------------------------------------------
      length |   57.20224   14.08047     4.06   0.000     29.13332    85.27115
       _cons |  -4584.899   2664.437    -1.72   0.090    -9896.357     726.559
------------------------------------------------------------------------------

. matrix table = r(table)

. tempname length_b

. tempname length_se

. scalar `length_b' = table[1,1]

. display `length_b' 57.202238
57.20223857.202238

. scalar `length_se' = table[2,1]

. display `length_b'
57.202238

. display "The coefficient of length in the regression is " `length_b' "."
The coefficient of length in the regression is 57.202238.

. display "The coefficient of length in the regression is " %3.2f `length_b' "
The coefficient of length in the regression is 57.20

. display "The standard error is " %3.2f `length_se' "."
The standard error is 14.08.

. matrix drop _all

. clear
```

CHAPTER 4

Variables, Variable Names, Value Label Names, Value Labels and Values

START BY LOADING THE auto dataset.

```
clear
sysuse auto


. clear

. sysuse auto
(1978 Automobile Data)
```

The variable foreign is categorical. Its characteristics can be displayed using the command codebook.

DOI: 10.1201/9781003483779-4

```
. codebook foreign

-------------------------------------------------------------------------------
foreign
-------------------------------------------------------------------------------

                  Type: Numeric (byte)
                 Label: origin

                 Range: [0,1]                         Units: 1
         Unique values: 2                         Missing .: 0/74

            Tabulation: Freq.   Numeric  Label
                           52         0  Domestic
                           22         1  Foreign

.
```

FIGURE 4.1

I. VARIABLE NAME

On the top left of the output is located the variable name "foreign" (without any quotation marks). This is the name that you use when you wish to identify the variable to Stata.

II. VARIABLE LABEL

On the top right-hand side of the output is the word "Car origin" (without any quotation marks). This is the variable label. It is often punctuated and can be used in output. Sometimes the variables can have rather obscure names for ease of computing. For example, serial data for ECGs may have variable names of ecg1 ecg2 ecg3 to represent data collected at three time points. The variable label, however, is likely to be more user-friendly and to be labelled "ECG at time 1", etc. However, this label would be cumbersome to manipulate in analyses, so the variable label is often only used for output.

III. VALUES OF A VARIABLE

The data that are held within the variable "foreign" are categorical and are composed of two values (0 and 1). This can be seen at the bottom of the output for codebook.

IV. VALUE LABEL NAME

These values have little meaning unless they have value names, and these are indicated next to the numbers, respectively (0 for Domestic and 1 for

Foreign). These two values and their labels are held in an entity called a value label name. The value label name for this variable ("foreign") is called "origin" (without any quotation marks). This is indicated by the output "label". The value label name is attached to the variable. You will need to know and manipulate all these entities in the next section when we start to use loops as the output will be used in reports.

V. VALUE LABELS

The values 0 and 1 for the variable have the names "Domestic" and "Foreign", respectively.

It may be helpful to construct a variable as practice.

Let's construct a variable called "pain" with a variable name of "Pain Experienced". The value label name will be called "levels_of_pain" and the values will range from 1 to 3 and have value labels of "Mild", "Moderate" and "Severe", respectively.

We will first of all clear Stata and create some test data for 20 observations.

We set a seed so that the output can be replicated later, if necessary.

```
clear
set obs 20
set seed 12345
gen pain = 20 * runiformint(0,3)


. clear

. set obs 20
number of observations (_N) was 0, now 20

. set seed 12345
```

To add a name to the variable:

```
label variable pain "Pain Experienced"

. label variable pain "Pain Experienced"
```

Just by looking at the variable window, you will see that the variable name has appeared. The next step is to define the value label name and simultaneously to enter the values for the data and their labels as below:

```
label define levels_of_pain 1 "Mild" 2 "Moderate" 3 "Severe"

. label define levels_of_pain 1 "Mild" 2 "Moderate" 3 "Severe"
```

Finally, you can now associate the value label to the variable:

```
label values pain levels_of_pain

. label values pain levels_of_pain
```

The results can be inspected by issuing the command **codebook**, and you can tabulate the variable with and without the value labels.

```
codebook
tabulate pain
tabulate pain, nol


. codebook pain

-------------------------------------------------------------------------------
pain
-------------------------------------------------------------------------------

                  type:  numeric (float)
                 label:  levels_of_pain, but 4 nonmissing values are not labeled

                 range:  [0,60]                       units:  10
         unique values:  4                        missing .:  0/20

            tabulation:  Freq.   Numeric  Label
                             7         0
                             7        20
                             5        40
                             1        60

. tabulate pain

       Pain |
Experienced |      Freq.     Percent        Cum.
------------+-----------------------------------
          0 |          7       35.00       35.00
         20 |          7       35.00       70.00
         40 |          5       25.00       95.00
         60 |          1        5.00      100.00
------------+-----------------------------------
      Total |         20      100.00

. tabulate pain, nol

       Pain |
Experienced |      Freq.     Percent        Cum.
------------+-----------------------------------
          0 |          7       35.00       35.00
         20 |          7       35.00       70.00
         40 |          5       25.00       95.00
         60 |          1        5.00      100.00
------------+-----------------------------------
      Total |         20      100.00
```

I would recommend you learn these definitions carefully; otherwise, the labelling in loops will be confusing.

CHAPTER 5

Loops

I. FOREACH

There are six types of ways in which to use foreach loops. You have already encountered some of these in the section on macros.

a. Using Foreach with a List

You can define a list and loop over it at the same time.

NOTE: This is the only time you will use "in" with "foreach", i.e. when you are creating a list to loop over. In all other instances in which you use "foreach", it will be followed by "of".

```
foreach i in "computer" "apple" "orange" {
display "i"
}.
```

b. Using Foreach with a Local Macro

You have encountered this previously, and a single exemplar suffices to illustrate.

```
local objects '"computer" "apple" "orange"'
'foreach i of local objects {
display' "i"
}
```

Note that when you use "in", you list the items individually, but when you use "of", you put them into a group (indicated by surrounding them with the appropriate quotation marks, backtick and apostrophe).

DOI: 10.1201/9781003483779-5

c. Using Foreach with a Global Macro

```
global objects '" "computer" "apple" "orange" "'

foreach i of global objects {
display '" 'i' "'
display '" "'i'" "'
}


. global objects '" "computer" "apple" "orange" "'


.
.     foreach i of global objects {
 2.
.     display '" 'i' "'
 3.     display '" "'i'" "'
 4.     }
computer
"computer"
apple
"apple"
orange
"orange"
```

d. Using Foreach with a Variable List

Suppose you wish to perform a statistical function on a list of variables.

```
clear
sysuse auto
foreach i of varlist price mpg {

display '" 'i' "'
summ 'i'
}

. clear

. sysuse auto
(1978 Automobile Data)

. foreach i of varlist price mpg {
  2.
. display '" 'i' "'
   3. summ 'i'
      4. }
 price

    Variable |        Obs        Mean    Std. Dev.       Min        Max
-------------+---------------------------------------------------------
       price |         74    6165.257    2949.496       3291      15906
 mpg

    Variable |        Obs        Mean    Std. Dev.       Min        Max
-------------+---------------------------------------------------------
         mpg |         74     21.2973    5.785503         12         41
```

A more elegant solution to naming the output would be to use the variable label rather than the variable itself.

```
sysuse auto
foreach i of varlist price mpg{
display "':variable label 'i' '"
display "************"
summ 'i'
di """
di ""
}
```

```
. sysuse auto
(1978 Automobile Data)

. foreach i of varlist price mpg{
  2. display " ':variable label 'i' '"
  3. display "************"
  4. summ 'i'
  5. di """
  6. di ""
  7. }
Price
************

    Variable |        Obs        Mean    Std. Dev.       Min        Max
-------------+---------------------------------------------------------
       price |         74    6165.257    2949.496       3291      15906

Mileage (mpg)
************

    Variable |        Obs        Mean    Std. Dev.       Min        Max
-------------+---------------------------------------------------------
         mpg |         74     21.2973    5.785503         12         41
```

Consider a categorical variable such as foreign. If you wished to look at the summary values for price by whether or not the car was domestic or foreign, you could do the following. It is possible to achieve this more elegantly using the command table, and we will cover that later in the course. For the moment, however, let's consider how to differentiate levels when using loops.

```
tabulate foreign
summ price if foreign == 0
summ price if foreign == 1
```

```
. tabulate foreign

   Car type |      Freq.     Percent        Cum.
------------+-----------------------------------
   Domestic |         52       70.27       70.27
    Foreign |         22       29.73      100.00
------------+-----------------------------------
      Total |         74      100.00

. summ price if foreign == 0

    Variable |        Obs        Mean    Std. Dev.       Min        Max
-------------+---------------------------------------------------------
       price |         52    6072.423    3097.104       3291      15906

. summ price if foreign == 1

    Variable |        Obs        Mean    Std. Dev.       Min        Max
-------------+---------------------------------------------------------
       price |         22    6384.682    2621.915       3748      12990
```

It is impossible to know what levels of foreign are unless you have previously tabulated foreign. You will need to label each summary with the value labels for each level as well as use the values themselves to restrict the summary function. In addition, it is necessary to discover the value label name itself.

```
levelsof foreign, miss local(levels)
local valuelabel: value label foreign
display "'valuelabel'"
foreach i of local levels{
display ":label 'valuelabel' 'i' "
display "*******"
summ price if foreign == 'i'
}
```

```
.

. levelsof foreign, miss local(levels)
0 1

. local valuelabel: value label foreign

. display  "" valuelabel ""
origin

. foreach i of local levels{
  2. display " :label 'valuelabel' 'i'  "
  3. display "*******"
  4. summ price if foreign == 'i'
  5. }
Domestic
*******

    Variable |        Obs        Mean    Std. Dev.       Min        Max
-------------+---------------------------------------------------------
       price |         52    6072.423    3097.104       3291      15906
Foreign
*******

    Variable |        Obs        Mean    Std. Dev.       Min        Max
-------------+---------------------------------------------------------
       price |         22    6384.682    2621.915       3748      12990
```

e. Using Foreach to Create New Variables

Foreach can also be used to create a series of similarly named variables in a loop. The syntax below should be fairly self-explanatory.

```
clear
set obs 20

foreach i of newlist ECG1-ECG8 {
gen 'i' = runiformint(1,8)
}

list in 1/5
```

```
. clear

. set obs 20
number of observations (_N) was 0, now 20

.
. foreach i of newlist ECG1-ECG8 {
  2. gen 'i' = runiformint(1,8)
  3. }

. list in 1/5
```

	ECG1	ECG2	ECG3	ECG4	ECG5	ECG6	ECG7	ECG8
1.	4	7	3	2	4	2	2	8
2.	6	8	6	7	6	8	6	1
3.	4	1	7	3	8	4	2	6
4.	6	2	8	8	6	8	3	1
5.	6	5	6	6	7	8	7	3

f. Using Foreach on a Numberlist

This loop allows you to create and loop over a numberlist simultaneously. You have encountered this previously. Another illustrative example is given here.

```
clear
foreach i of numlist 1 8/12 14(6)32 134 {
display "' i '"
}

. clear

. foreach i of numlist 1 8/12 14(6)32 134 {
  2. display "'i'"
  3. }
1
8
9
10
11
12
14
20
26
32
134
```

II. FORVALUES

This is a very efficient way of looping over a list of numbers (see an alternative method in the example above). However, it is not quite as flexible as using a numlist in foreach. In the first example, the numbers 8 to 12 are displayed, and in the second, the numbers from 10 to 30 in steps of 4 are displayed.

```
forvalues i = 8/12{
display "'i'"
}

forvalues i = 4 10 : 30{
display 'i'
}

. forvalues i = 8/12{
  2. display "'i'"
  3. }
8
9
10
11
12

.
. forvalues i = 4 10 : 30{
  2. display 'i'
  3. }
4
10
16
22
28
```

III. IF, ELSE AND ELSE IF

The next four commands are conditional on the outcome of the statement that precedes the loop itself. You have already encountered this in the example of using time.

```
if c(current_time) < "12:00:00" {
local greeting "Good Morning"
}

else if c(current_time) >= "12:00:00" & c(current_time) < "17:00:00" {
local greeting "Good Afternoon"
}

else if c(current_time) >= "17:00:00" & c(current_time) < "19:00:00" {
local greeting "Good Evening"
}

else{
local greeting "Good Night Irene"
}

display "`greeting'"

. if c(current_time) < "12:00:00" {
. local greeting "Good Morning"
. }
.
. else if c(current_time) >= "12:00:00" & c(current_time) < "17:00:00" {
. local greeting "Good Afternoon"
. }

.
. else if c(current_time) >= "17:00:00" & c(current_time) < "19:00:00"{
. local greeting "Good Evening"
. }

.
. else{
. local greeting "Good Night Irene"
. }

.

.
. display "`greeting'"
Good Afternoon
```

IV. WHILE

This command is most frequently encountered when writing Stata programs. It is included for completeness here, but you may wish to skip over this section.

The only syntax that is new is that the local i changes at every loop and serves as a counter. If you are keen to use this command, please refer to the Stata help files.

CHAPTER 6

Append, Merge and Collapse

THESE THREE COMMANDS are frequently encountered together. Merge is used when we wish to add variables from one dataset to another. Append is used when we wish to add observations to the existing dataset. Collapse is used to change the dataset so that it now includes a summary measure of one (or more) of the existing variables.

I. MERGE

A bit of terminology: the "Master" dataset is the term used by Stata to identify the dataset that is in memory. The observations from the dataset that you are joining to the Master are termed "using" by Stata, which is very confusing to my mind as you are using both datasets to produce a new dataset with combined values. But leave that aside.

DOI: 10.1201/9781003483779-6

Here is how this is done:

```
use "`c(pwd)'/Data_In/Stata_Data/odd.dta", clear
merge 1:1 id using "`c(pwd)'/Data_In/Stata_Data/even.dta"
```

```
. use "`c(pwd)'/Data_In/Stata_Data/odd.dta", clear
(First five odd numbers)

. merge 1:1 id using "`c(pwd)'/Data_In/Stata_Data/even.dta"

    Result                           # of obs.
    -----------------------------------------
    not matched                             8
        from master                         5  (_merge==1)
        from using                          3  (_merge==2)

    matched                                 0  (_merge==3)
    -----------------------------------------

.
```

Note that Stata automatically includes a variable called "_merge" which displays information about the merge. While this can be helpful, you often don't want this variable in the final dataset, and you can stop Stata from doing this by using the option nogen as here:

```
use "`c(pwd)'/Data_In/Stata_Data/odd.dta", clear
merge 1:1 id using "`c(pwd)'/Data_In/Stata_Data/even.dta", nogen
```

```
. merge 1:1 id using "`c(pwd)'/Data_In/Stata_Data/even.dta", nogen

    Result                           # of obs.
    -----------------------------------------
    not matched                             8
        from master                         5
        from using                          3

    matched                                 0
    -----------------------------------------

.
```

II. APPEND

You often wish to append several datasets. Very large electronic health data are stored in several files which you need to append to produce a final analysis dataset. It's best to do this in a loop. First of all, create a local macro with the names of the datasets you wish to append. Then randomly load one of these and drop all the observations. That way, you end upf with the variables and the variable names, so you can append all the datasets on to this one.

III. COLLAPSE

This command is used to create summary measures on an outcome based on another variable. It is very frequently encountered in electronic health record analyses.

Let's load the dataset provided by Stata of Grade Point Averages (GPA). https://www.stata-press.com/data/r17/class10.dta

```
use "`c(pwd)'/Data_In/Stata_Data/gpa.dta", clear
describe


. use "`c(pwd)'/Data_In/Stata_Data/gpa.dta", clear

. describe

Contains data from c:\EHR_Course/Data_In/Stata_Data/gpa.dta
  obs:            12


 vars:             4                    18 Apr 2019 15:59
 size:           120
--------------------------------------------------------------------------------------
                storage   display     value
variable name    type      format      label      variable label
--------------------------------------------------------------------------------------
gpa             float     %9.0g                  GPS for the year
hour            int       %9.0g                  Total academic hours
year            int       %9.0g      year_label
                                                 Year
number          int       %9.0g                  Number of Students
--------------------------------------------------------------------------------------
Sorted by: year
```

You wish to find out the average GPA for each year. You could display these values using Stata's table function. We will explore the functions table and tabulate in greater depth later in the book. The syntax is that the categories of the output appear on the right-hand side of the table. This is followed by a comma, and then the contents of the rest of the table are indicated by the letter "c" and in the parenthesis the summary statistic is followed by the variable. You can have more than one variable if you wish. The format option has been explained previously. The column headings for summary statistics for continuous variables are not acceptable in terms of presentation for publications, so this needs to be changed by hand at the editing stage. Stata does not have the option to change column headings at this stage of the analysis. (Please note that this syntax is only allowed up to Stata 17.) The syntax for making more complicated (publication ready) tables is given in the chapter on Automated Reporting. This syntax is given for those of you using Stata 17 or earlier versions which support the table command.

```
table year, c(mean gpa) format (%3.2fc)

.
. table year, c(mean gpa) format (%3.2fc)

-------------------------
        Year | mean(gpa)
-------------+-----------
    Freshman |      2.90
   Sophomore |      3.07
      Junior |      3.07
      Senior |      3.15
-------------------------

.
end of do-file
```

Let's take a trivial example using the auto dataset.

Let's suppose you wanted to look at the relationship between mpg and weight adjusting for mean trunk space for foreign and domestic vehicles.

Let's load the dataset to begin with and refamiliarise ourselves with the variables.

```
sysuse auto, clear

. sysuse auto, clear
(1978 Automobile Data)
```

The collapse command is demonstrated below and is fairly intuitive. The syntax of "trunk = mean_trunk" indicates to Stata that it should produce the mean trunk size for each level of the variable "foreign" and create a new variable called "mean_trunk". Otherwise, it creates a variable called "trunk", and you have no idea what the collapse summary statistic used was by looking at the name.

```
collapse (mean) mean_trunk=trunk, by (foreign)
list

. collapse (mean) mean_trunk=trunk, by (foreign)

. list

     +---------------------+
     |  foreign   mean_t~k |
     |---------------------|
  1. | Domestic      14.75 |
  2. |  Foreign    11.4091 |
     +---------------------+
```

Now you wish to merge this dataset back on to the main dataset, so these variables are available for the main regress command. We will accomplish this below. You will encounter two new Stata commands: preserve and restore. These commands occur in pairs. Once you issue the command "preserve", Stata will keep a snapshot of the dataset as it is at the time you issue the command. If the program subsequently breaks or it encounters the command "restore", it will replace the contents of its display with the preserved dataset without alerting you to the fact that the dataset is being restored or seeking your confirmation.

```
sysuse auto, clear
preserve
collapse (mean) mean_trunk=trunk, by (foreign)
tempfile mean_trunk
save `mean_trunk', replace
restore
merge m:1 foreign using `mean_trunk', nogen


. sysuse auto, clear
(1978 Automobile Data)

. preserve

. collapse (mean) mean_trunk=trunk, by (foreign)

. tempfile mean_trunk

. save `mean_trunk', replace

. restore

. merge m:1 foreign using `mean_trunk', nogen
(label origin already defined)


    Result                           # of obs.
    -----------------------------------------
    not matched                              0
    matched                                 74
    -----------------------------------------
```

We preserve the original dataset, collapse to create the "mean_trunk" variable, save this to a temporary dataset, restore the original dataset and merge the variable we wish back on.

However, this means we have created a derived variable in our original dataset. We could remember to delete this later at the end of the analysis, but it's far better never to adulterate your original data. In the iteration of the analysis below, we will create a temporary file, carry out the analysis and restore our original data.

```
sysuse auto, clear
preserve
collapse (mean) mean_trunk =trunk, by (foreign)
tempfile mean_trunk
save `mean_trunk', replace
restore
preserve
merge m:1 foreign using `mean_trunk', nogen
regress mpg weigh mean_trunk
restore
```

```
. sysuse auto, clear
(1978 Automobile Data)

. preserve

. collapse (mean) mean_trunk =trunk, by (foreign)

. tempfile mean_trunk

. save `mean_trunk', replace

. restore

. preserve

. merge m:1 foreign using `mean_trunk', nogen
(label origin already defined)

    Result                           # of obs.
    -----------------------------------------
    not matched                             0
    matched                                74
    -----------------------------------------

. regress mpg weigh mean_trunk

      Source |       SS           df       MS      Number of obs   =        74
-------------+----------------------------------   F(2, 71)        =     69.75
       Model |   1619.2877         2  809.643849   Prob > F        =    0.0000
    Residual |  824.171761        71   11.608053   R-squared       =    0.6627
-------------+----------------------------------   Adj R-squared   =    0.6532
       Total |  2443.45946        73  33.4720474   Root MSE        =    3.4071

------------------------------------------------------------------------------
         mpg |      Coef.   Std. Err.      t    P>|t|     [95% Conf. Interval]
-------------+----------------------------------------------------------------
      weight |  -.0065879   .0006371   -10.34   0.000    -.0078583   -.0053175
  mean_trunk |   .4938863   .3220663     1.53   0.130    -.1482956    1.136068
       _cons |   34.39488   3.658144     9.40   0.000     27.10075    41.68901
------------------------------------------------------------------------------
```

CHAPTER 7

Reshape

I. FROM WIDE TO LONG FORMATS

Data that contain repeated observations for a given individual can be formatted in either "wide" or "long" format. It's easier and more intuitive to enter data into a dataset in "wide" format. In this format, the repeated observations are entered horizontally usually in columns of data that are adjacent to the repeated observations of a given variable (e.g. ECG_1, ECG_2, ECG_3, etc.). This type of format is also useful for counting row totals, for identifying individuals with missing data, etc.

Analysis of these datasets often requires that the data be in "long" format, which means that repeated observations are in subsequent rows, not columns. It's when the data are in this format that you can use _n and N commands. These will be covered later in the course but are essential commands in the analysis of repeated measurement data (where there are repeated observations for any given individual).

Therefore, it is an essential skill to be able to easily reformat data between these two dataset types.

It's best to illustrate the concepts of wide and long data by looking at actual data in these formats. Let's start with wide data as this is the format in which you are most likely to initially encounter your dataset for analysis. These data are located here:

http://www.stata-press.com/data/r15/reshapel.dta

DOI: 10.1201/9781003483779-7

```
use "`c(pwd)'/Data_In/Stata_Data/income_wide.dta", clear
list

.
. use "`c(pwd)'/Data_In/Stata_Data/income_wide.dta", clear

. list

     +--------------------------------------------------------------------------------+
     | id      sex   inc80   inc81   inc82          ue80          ue81          ue82 |
     |--------------------------------------------------------------------------------|
  1. |  1   Female   5,000   5,500   6,000      Employed    Unemployed      Employed |
  2. |  2     Male   2,000   2,200   3,300    Unemployed      Employed      Employed |
  3. |  3   Female   3,000   2,000   1,000      Employed      Employed    Unemployed |
     +--------------------------------------------------------------------------------+
```

Browse the data and become a bit more familiar with the variables. You will notice that these data are given for three individuals. The participant's sex is also given. The variables of income and unemployment status are repeatedly recorded, and we will practice reshaping these data into long format. Note that the stubs of the repeated measurements ("inc …" and "ue …") are the same for each of the two sets of repeated measurements. If you are unfortunate enough to inherit a dataset where this is not the case then there is little alternative but to make sure the names fit this format. Stata identifies repeated measurements by this stub and uses the stub to name the columns in the long format.

II. FROM LONG TO WIDE FORMATS

Let's look at these data in long format.

```
use "`c(pwd)'/Data_In/Stata_Data/income_long.dta", clear
list

     +------------------------------------------+
     | id   year      sex     inc           ue |
     |------------------------------------------|
  1. |  1     80   Female   5,000     Employed |
  2. |  1     81   Female   5,500   Unemployed |
  3. |  1     82   Female   6,000     Employed |
  4. |  2     80     Male   2,000   Unemployed |
  5. |  2     81     Male   2,200     Employed |
     |------------------------------------------|
  6. |  2     82     Male   3,300     Employed |
  7. |  3     80   Female   3,000     Employed |
  8. |  3     81   Female   2,000     Employed |
  9. |  3     82   Female   1,000   Unemployed |
     +------------------------------------------+
```

Note that there is no longer one observation per individual but one row per observation. The repeat observations are now in sequential rows (instead of columns). In particular, note that Stata has created an entirely new variable that records the units of interval between the two measurements. This is the variable "year", and when reshaping from wide to long, you will need to specify this variable.

Stata has taken the serial columns of income and unemployment status and collapsed each of these sets of variables into columns. The name of the column is the stub, which you identified earlier for each of the two sets of variables. Since the gender and ID number are unchanged between serial observations, they are replicated unchanged by Stata in the subsequent rows for each individual.

To change from wide to long format, employ the following syntax.

```
use "`c(pwd)'/Data_In/Stata_Data/income_wide.dta" , clear
reshape long ue inc, i(id) j(year)
```

```
. reshape long ue inc, i(id) j(year)
(note: j = 80 81 82)

Data                               wide   ->   long
-----------------------------------------------------------------------------
Number of obs.                        3   ->      9
Number of variables                   8   ->      5
j variable (3 values)                     ->   year
xij variables:
                         ue80 ue81 ue82   ->   ue
                      inc80 inc81 inc82   ->   inc
-----------------------------------------------------------------------------

. list
```

	id	year	sex	inc	ue
1.	1	80	Female	5,000	Employed
2.	1	81	Female	5,500	Unemployed
3.	1	82	Female	6,000	Employed
4.	2	80	Male	2,000	Unemployed
5.	2	81	Male	2,200	Employed
6.	2	82	Male	3,300	Employed
7.	3	80	Female	3,000	Employed
8.	3	81	Female	2,000	Employed
9.	3	82	Female	1,000	Unemployed

The syntax is broken down as follows: "reshape long" is obvious, followed by the variables that you wish to have in long format, i represents the identifier for each individual and j is the name of the new variable which will hold the time measurement.

Note that many of your variable names are lost for the repeated measurements, and you will need to recreate these once the data are in the long format.

Stata assumes that any variable not listed in the reshape command is not varying and so replicates the values for each row in the long format.

To change from wide back to long, employ the following syntax.

reshape wide

```
. reshape wide
(note: j = 80 81 82)

Data                               long   ->   wide
-----------------------------------------------------------------------------
Number of obs.                        9   ->       3
Number of variables                   5   ->       8
j variable (3 values)              year   ->   (dropped)
xij variables:
                                     ue   ->   ue80 ue81 ue82
                                    inc   ->   inc80 inc81 inc82
-----------------------------------------------------------------------------

. list

     +-----------------------------------------------------------------------------------------+
     | id   inc80          ue80   inc81          ue81   inc82          ue82      sex |
     |-----------------------------------------------------------------------------------------|
  1. |  1   5,000      Employed   5,500    Unemployed   6,000      Employed   Female |
  2. |  2   2,000    Unemployed   2,200      Employed   3,300      Employed     Male |
  3. |  3   3,000      Employed   2,000      Employed   1,000    Unemployed   Female |
     +-----------------------------------------------------------------------------------------+
```

Let's import these data in the long format and reshape them to the wide format.

```
use "'c(pwd)'/Data_In/Stata_Data/income_long.dta" , clear
reshape wide ue inc, i(id) j(year)
list
```

```
. use "'c(pwd)'/Data_In/Stata_Data/income_long.dta", clear

. reshape wide ue inc, i(id) j(year)
(note: j = 80 81 82)

Data                               long   ->   wide
-----------------------------------------------------------------------------
Number of obs.                        9   ->      3
Number of variables                   5   ->      8
j variable (3 values)              year   ->   (dropped)
xij variables:
                                     ue   ->   ue80 ue81 ue82
                                    inc   ->   inc80 inc81 inc82
-----------------------------------------------------------------------------

. list

     +----------------------------------------------------------------------------------+
     | id   inc80         ue80   inc81         ue81   inc82          ue82      sex |
     |----------------------------------------------------------------------------------|
  1. |  1   5,000     Employed   5,500   Unemployed   6,000      Employed   Female |
  2. |  2   2,000   Unemployed   2,200     Employed   3,300      Employed     Male |
  3. |  3   3,000     Employed   2,000     Employed   1,000    Unemployed   Female |
     +----------------------------------------------------------------------------------+
```

CHAPTER 8

Dates

HANDLING DATES is not straightforward. The Stata helpfile can be called up using “help datetime”.

The most common manipulations of date and time will be covered here, but this topic is by no means covered exhaustively in this introductory chapter.

Dates displayed in Stata that approximate something familiar (such as “1 Jan 2018” or “01/01/208”) are termed HRF (Human Readable Form). This is not the format in which Stata has stored the data but simply the format in which it is displayed so humans can more easily understand the stored data. The storage form that Stata uses to hold data in a way that it understands and can manipulate is called “SIF” (Stata Internal Form). Honestly. I didn’t make up these acronyms, however imaginative you might find them. SIFs hold the data as an integer, which represents the number of milliseconds between the date you have entered and the arbitrary date of 1 January 1960.

DOI: 10.1201/9781003483779-8

I. HOW TO ENTER DATES INTO STATA

Let's start with an empty dataset and create one column of empty observations for a string variable named date.

```
clear
set obs 3
gen date_HRF = ""


. clear

. set obs 3
number of observations (_N) was 0, now 3

. gen date_HRF = ""
(3 missing values generated)
```

Let's enter a date.

```
replace date_HRF = "28 June 1851" in 1
replace date_HRF = "17 Jan 1999" in 2
replace date_HRF = "01 January 1960" in 3
list


. replace date_HRF = "28 June 1851"
variable date_HRF was str1 now str12
(3 real changes made)

. replace date_HRF = "17 Jan 1999" in 2
(1 real change made)

. replace date_HRF = "01 January 1960" in 3
variable date_HRF was str12 now str15
(1 real change made)

. list

     +-----------------+
     |        date_HRF |
     |-----------------|
  1. |    28 June 1851 |
  2. |     17 Jan 1999 |
  3. | 01 January 1960 |
     +-----------------+
```

To Stata, this entry is a string, and Stata cannot manipulate it in its current state. Say, for example, you wanted to know the time between today's date and this date, Stata could only do this manipulation if the date entered was in SIF.

To convert this date to SIF, proceed as follows:

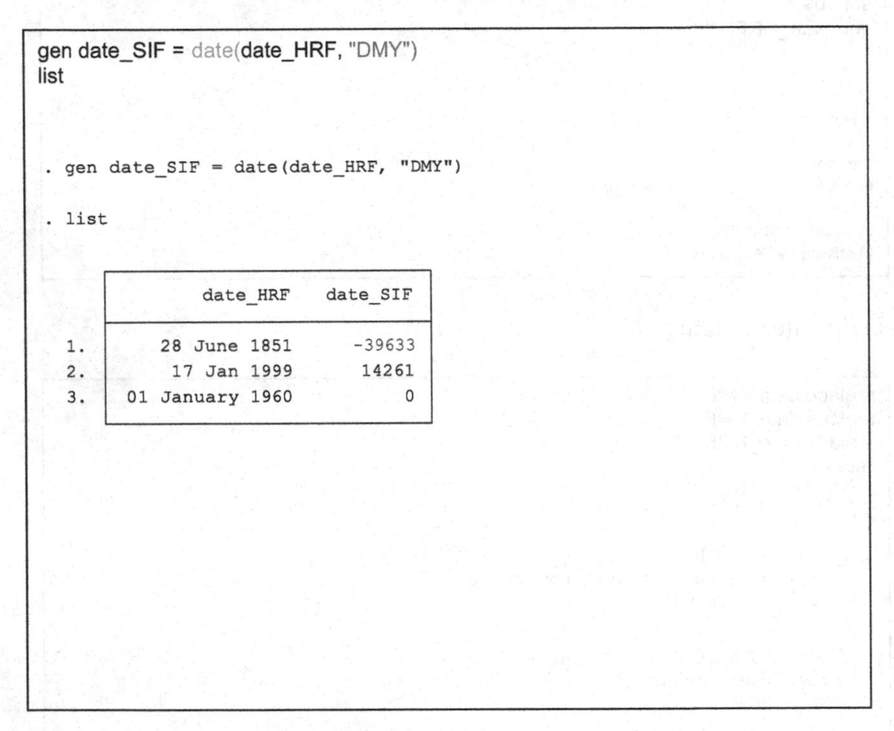

```
gen date_SIF = date(date_HRF, "DMY")
list

. gen date_SIF = date(date_HRF, "DMY")

. list

     +--------------------------------+
     |        date_HRF     date_SIF   |
     |--------------------------------|
  1. |    28 June 1851       -39633   |
  2. |     17 Jan 1999        14261   |
  3. | 01 January 1960            0   |
     +--------------------------------+
```

The first date is a negative number because it has occurred before 1 January 1960. The second is positive, as it occurs after the Stata date of 01 January 1960. The last is 0 for obvious reasons.

These numbers are not very helpful to work with, so you will now apply a "mask" to the numbers so that they are formatted and displayed in a manner that humans can interpret.

II. HOW TO FORMAT SIF TO HRF

```
format date_SIF %d
list

.         format date_SIF %d

.         list

     +-----------------------------+
     |       date_HRF     date_SIF |
     |-----------------------------|
  1. |   28 June 1851    28jun1851 |
  2. |    17 Jan 1999    17jan1999 |
  3. | 01 January 1960   01jan1960 |
     +-----------------------------+
```

Browse the data and observe that date_HRF and date_SIF appear superficially similar. However, date_SIF is only displayed as text. It is in fact stored and manipulated as an integer, while date_HRF is a string. You can enter text directly into Stata and tell it that it's a date, so it's stored correctly.

```
clear
set obs 1
gen date = date("31 October 2014", "DMY")
format %dDD_Month_CCYY date
list in 1

. clear

. set obs 1
number of observations(_N) was 0, now 1

. gen date = date("31 October 2014", "DMY")

. format %dDD_Month_CCYY date

. list in 1

     +-----------------+
     |            date |
     |-----------------|
  1. | 31 October 2014 |
```

Look at the format command and try to understand what each element of the format string is doing. You can change "Month" to "Mon", "DD" to "dd" "CCYY" to "YY", etc., until you get the type of format you're comfortable with. The one used in the illustration is frequently encountered and has the advantage of being easily read and not prone to being misinterpreted. Be cautious about displaying dates with only numbers as in the United States the month comes before the day. For example, 01/04/2003 could be interpreted either as 1st of April or 4th of January. It is recommended therefore always to display the month in words to avoid confusion. In the syntax above, replacing "DD" with "dd" drops any leading zeros in the displayed date. Abbreviating the command "Month" to "Mon" abbreviates the month displayed to three letters. Do not ever change the uppercase of either C or Y to lowercase. If you do not use the "CC" command, then the first two digits of a four digit year will be dropped.

CHAPTER 9

Bits and Bobs

THESE COMMANDS DON'T EASILY FIT into the headings of the previous chapters so are presented here. I have chosen to include them simply because of their utility. As you become experienced in programming, no doubt you will acquire additional commands that you will find invaluable. For the beginner, I think these should suffice.

I. SORT, GSORT, BY AND BYSORT

a. Sort

Sort does exactly what you would expect it to. It sorts invariably from smaller to larger (if the variable is numeric) or from A to Z (if the variable is a string).

Sort the dataset by whether or not the car is foreign or imported, then by weight, then by price.

DOI: 10.1201/9781003483779-9

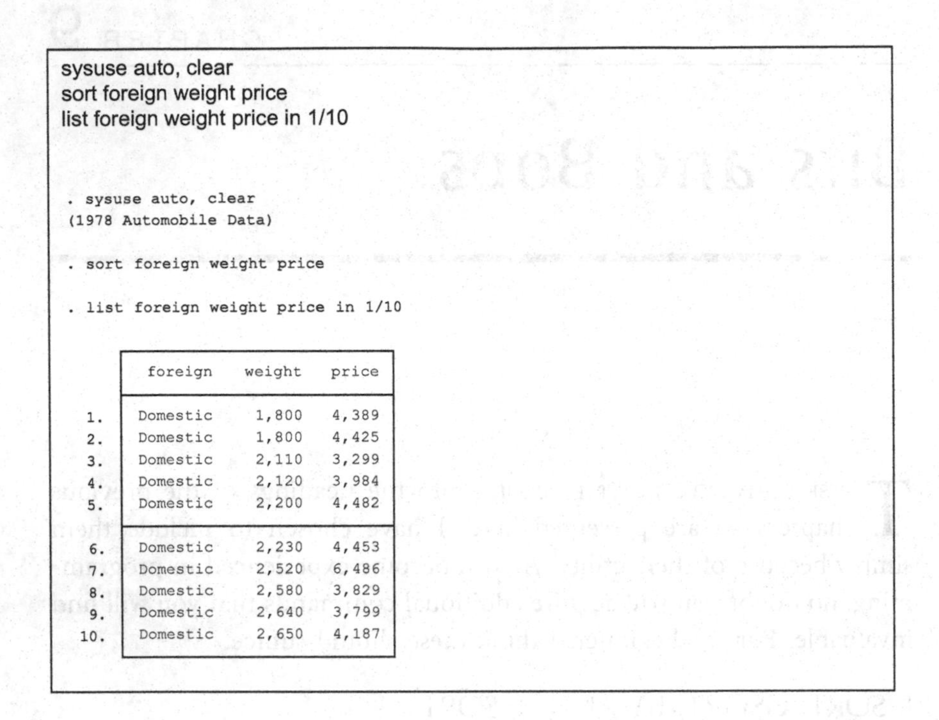

```
sysuse auto, clear
sort foreign weight price
list foreign weight price in 1/10
```

```
. sysuse auto, clear
(1978 Automobile Data)

. sort foreign weight price

. list foreign weight price in 1/10
```

	foreign	weight	price
1.	Domestic	1,800	4,389
2.	Domestic	1,800	4,425
3.	Domestic	2,110	3,299
4.	Domestic	2,120	3,984
5.	Domestic	2,200	4,482
6.	Domestic	2,230	4,453
7.	Domestic	2,520	6,486
8.	Domestic	2,580	3,829
9.	Domestic	2,640	3,799
10.	Domestic	2,650	4,187

Note in lines 1 and 2 that the contents are identical for the origin and weight.

b. gsort

gsort allows you to alter the direction of sorting. To sort the auto dataset for the same three variables in descending order:

```
gsort -foreign -weight -price
list foreign weight price in 1/10

. gsort -foreign -weight -price

. list foreign weight price in 1/10
```

	foreign	weight	price
1.	Foreign	3,420	12,990
2.	Foreign	3,170	11,995
3.	Foreign	2,830	9,690
4.	Foreign	2,750	8,129
5.	Foreign	2,670	5,719
6.	Foreign	2,650	9,735
7.	Foreign	2,410	5,899
8.	Foreign	2,370	6,229
9.	Foreign	2,280	5,079
10.	Foreign	2,240	5,799

c. By and bysort

The command "by" is always followed by a full colon. By allows you to repeat commands over a range of sets of variables.

If you wish to find the mean weight of car by whether or not it was foreign or domestic, you could use the table command (this syntax works up to Stata 17):

```
table foreign, c(mean weight)

. table foreign, c(mean weight)
```

Car type	mean(weight)
Domestic	3,317.1
Foreign	2,315.9

But, if you wished these numbers to be entered as a variable in the dataset so you could use them in a subsequent estimation command, you could:

```
. sysuse auto, clear
(1978 automobile data)

. sort foreign

.
. by foreign: egen mean_wt = mean(weight)

. by foreign: egen mean_lt = mean(length)

. by foreign: egen mean_trn = mean(turn)

.
. list  foreign mean* in 1/20, noobs abb(20) sepby(foreign)
```

foreign	mean_wt	mean_lt	mean_trn
Domestic	3317.115	196.1346	41.44231
Domestic	3317.115	196.1346	41.44231
Domestic	3317.115	196.1346	41.44231
Domestic	3317.115	196.1346	41.44231
Domestic	3317.115	196.1346	41.44231
Domestic	3317.115	196.1346	41.44231
Domestic	3317.115	196.1346	41.44231
Domestic	3317.115	196.1346	41.44231
Domestic	3317.115	196.1346	41.44231
Domestic	3317.115	196.1346	41.44231
Domestic	3317.115	196.1346	41.44231
Domestic	3317.115	196.1346	41.44231
Domestic	3317.115	196.1346	41.44231
Domestic	3317.115	196.1346	41.44231
Domestic	3317.115	196.1346	41.44231
Domestic	3317.115	196.1346	41.44231
Domestic	3317.115	196.1346	41.44231
Domestic	3317.115	196.1346	41.44231
Domestic	3317.115	196.1346	41.44231
Domestic	3317.115	196.1346	41.44231

You have to sort data before you can use the "by" command. This can be done in two steps as in the first example. In the second step, bysort uses the variable foreign for "by" as well as sorts on this variable. In the third example, you indicate "by" and "sort" commands separately but in one line.

You have now encountered the egen command. *egen* stands for "extended generate". This function will be covered later in the course.

You could also do this for two or more variables. In this case, you are generating the mean weight of each car by origin as well as by rep78 category.

```
sysuse auto, clear
sort foreign rep78
by foreign rep78: egen mean_wt1 = mean(weight)
bysort foreign rep78 : egen mean_w2 = mean(weight)
by foreign rep78, sort:egen mean_wt3 = mean(weight)
list foreign rep78 weight mean* in 1/20
```

```
. sysuse auto, clear
(1978 Automobile Data)

. sort foreign rep78

. by foreign rep78: egen mean_wt1 = mean(weight)

. bysort foreign rep78 : egen mean_w2 = mean(weight)

. by foreign rep78, sort:egen mean_wt3 = mean(weight)

. list foreign rep78 weight mean* in 1/20
```

	foreign	rep78	weight	mean_wt1	mean_w2	mean_wt3
1.	Domestic	1	3,470	3100	3100	3100
2.	Domestic	1	2,730	3100	3100	3100
3.	Domestic	2	3,220	3353.75	3353.75	3353.75
4.	Domestic	2	2,690	3353.75	3353.75	3353.75
5.	Domestic	2	3,330	3353.75	3353.75	3353.75
6.	Domestic	2	2,750	3353.75	3353.75	3353.75
7.	Domestic	2	3,600	3353.75	3353.75	3353.75
8.	Domestic	2	3,740	3353.75	3353.75	3353.75
9.	Domestic	2	3,600	3353.75	3353.75	3353.75
10.	Domestic	2	3,900	3353.75	3353.75	3353.75
11.	Domestic	3	3,670	3442.222	3442.222	3442.222
12.	Domestic	3	3,210	3442.222	3442.222	3442.222
13.	Domestic	3	3,300	3442.222	3442.222	3442.222
14.	Domestic	3	3,310	3442.222	3442.222	3442.222
15.	Domestic	3	4,030	3442.222	3442.222	3442.222
16.	Domestic	3	3,720	3442.222	3442.222	3442.222
17.	Domestic	3	2,200	3442.222	3442.222	3442.222
18.	Domestic	3	3,430	3442.222	3442.222	3442.222
19.	Domestic	3	3,250	3442.222	3442.222	3442.222
20.	Domestic	3	2,930	3442.222	3442.222	3442.222

In the event you only wanted to sort the data by origin and rep78, but wished only to find the mean weight by origin, you would enclose the variable rep78 in brackets.

```
sysuse auto, clear
bysort foreign (rep78): egen mean_wt= mean(weight)
list foreign rep78 weight mean* in 1/20
```

```
. sysuse auto, clear
(1978 Automobile Data)

. bysort foreign (rep78): egen mean_wt= mean(weight)

. list foreign rep78 weight mean* in 1/20

     +------------------------------------------+
     |  foreign   rep78   weight     mean_wt    |
     |------------------------------------------|
  1. | Domestic       1    3,470    3317.115    |
  2. | Domestic       1    2,730    3317.115    |
  3. | Domestic       2    3,220    3317.115    |
  4. | Domestic       2    3,900    3317.115    |
  5. | Domestic       2    3,600    3317.115    |
     |------------------------------------------|
  6. | Domestic       2    3,330    3317.115    |
  7. | Domestic       2    2,690    3317.115    |
  8. | Domestic       2    3,740    3317.115    |
  9. | Domestic       2    2,750    3317.115    |
 10. | Domestic       2    3,600    3317.115    |
     |------------------------------------------|
 11. | Domestic       3    3,260    3317.115    |
 12. | Domestic       3    3,310    3317.115    |
 13. | Domestic       3    2,650    3317.115    |
 14. | Domestic       3    2,110    3317.115    |
 15. | Domestic       3    3,720    3317.115    |
     |------------------------------------------|
 16. | Domestic       3    3,430    3317.115    |
 17. | Domestic       3    4,330    3317.115    |
 18. | Domestic       3    3,370    3317.115    |
 19. | Domestic       3    3,400    3317.115    |
 20. | Domestic       3    3,880    3317.115    |
```

An alternative syntax would be:

```
sysuse auto, clear
by foreign (rep78), sort: egen mean_wt= mean(weight)
list foreign rep78 weight mean* in 1/20

. sysuse auto, clear
(1978 Automobile Data)

. by foreign (rep78), sort: egen mean_wt= mean(weight)

. list foreign rep78 weight mean* in 1/20

     +------------------------------------------+
     |  foreign   rep78   weight      mean_wt   |
     |------------------------------------------|
  1. | Domestic       1    3,470     3317.115   |
  2. | Domestic       1    2,730     3317.115   |
  3. | Domestic       2    3,900     3317.115   |
  4. | Domestic       2    2,690     3317.115   |
  5. | Domestic       2    3,330     3317.115   |
     |------------------------------------------|
  6. | Domestic       2    3,600     3317.115   |
  7. | Domestic       2    2,750     3317.115   |
  8. | Domestic       2    3,600     3317.115   |
  9. | Domestic       2    3,220     3317.115   |
 10. | Domestic       2    3,740     3317.115   |
     |------------------------------------------|
 11. | Domestic       3    3,350     3317.115   |
 12. | Domestic       3    2,110     3317.115   |
 13. | Domestic       3    3,300     3317.115   |
 14. | Domestic       3    3,310     3317.115   |
 15. | Domestic       3    3,720     3317.115   |
     |------------------------------------------|
 16. | Domestic       3    3,260     3317.115   |
 17. | Domestic       3    3,200     3317.115   |
 18. | Domestic       3    4,720     3317.115   |
 19. | Domestic       3    2,830     3317.115   |
 20. | Domestic       3    3,210     3317.115   |
     +------------------------------------------+
```

Note that you have now created a new variable in the dataset, and this is not good programming practice to adulterate your original data. If, for example, you wished to perform a regression estimation, you could create a temporary variable, perform the regression and obtain the results. The temporary variable would then disappear at the end of the analysis, and your original data would be left undisturbed.

```
sysuse auto, clear
tempvar mean_wt
bysort foreign (rep78): egen `mean_wt' = mean(weight)
codebook `mean_wt'
```

```
. sysuse auto, clear
(1978 Automobile Data)

. tempvar mean_wt

. bysort foreign (rep78): egen `mean_wt' = mean(weight)

. codebook `mean_wt'

-------------------------------------------------------------------------------
__000000
-------------------------------------------------------------------------------

                  type:  numeric (float)

                 range:  [2315.9092,3317.1155]        units:  .0001
         unique values:  2                        missing .:  0/74

            tabulation:  Freq.  Value
                            22  2315.9092
                            52  3317.1155
```

II. GEN AND EGEN

You have previously encountered the command gen. This is simply used to generate a new variable and should be intuitive.

egen is an extended command for gen, and there are a lot of egen commands you may find helpful. The Stata help files are particularly helpful.

III. TABLE AND TABULATE

tabulate will do exactly this for two categorical variables, plus you can test the association. The most commonly used test is chi2.

Load a sample dataset of food preferences by gender and test if there is an association:

```
use "`c(pwd)'/Data_In/Stata_Data/categorical.dta", clear
tabulate gender food, chi2
```

```
. use "`c(pwd)'/Data_In/Stata_Data/categorical.dta", clear

. tabulate gender food, chi2

           |       Food Type
    Gender |     Salty      Sweet |     Total
-----------+----------------------+----------
      Girl |        30         29 |        59
       Boy |        23         18 |        41
-----------+----------------------+----------
     Total |        53         47 |       100

          Pearson chi2(1) =   0.2677   Pr = 0.605

.
```

table will allow you to summarise one variable against a categorical one (using Stata version 17).

Summarise the weight of cars by origin.

```
sysuse auto, clear
table foreign, c(n weight min weight max weight mean weight median weight)
```

```
. sysuse auto, clear
(1978 Automobile Data)

. table foreign, c(n weight min weight max weight mean weight median weight)
```

Car type	N(weight)	min(weight)	max(weight)	mean(weight)	med(weight)
Domestic	52	1,800	4,840	3,317.1	3,360
Foreign	22	1,760	3,420	2,315.9	2,180

III. ORDER AND SORT

These terms can be very confusing if you also program in R as they mean very different things in R.

Order is used to change the order of the variable names in the dataset. Sort is used to order the observations from smallest to largest.

IV. DISPLAYING LINES AND OTHER REPETITIVE SYMBOLS

You may wish to display a line across the page or enter several empty lines so as to separate your output.

_dup is invaluable.

To display a line that is composed of 30 consecutive iterations of the character use the command "_". You can, obviously, replace the character with any you wish.

```
display _dup(30) "_"


. display _dup(30) "_"
______________________________

.
```

To leave a space between outputs, use the ASCII character number for character return (13). You can enter any ASCII number, and it will be displayed.

```
display _char(13)
display "x"
display _char(13)
display "X"




. display _char(13)



. display "x"
x

. display _char(13)



. display "X"
X
```

V. _N & _N

_n is used to generate a sequence of numbers of observations. This can be done by subcategorising within the data. _N indicates the total number in each category (if they exist). It's easier to explain these concepts using an example.

Obtain the second largest weights from the auto dataset by origin and display them in appropriate sentences.

```
sysuse auto, clear
sort foreign weight
levelsof foreign, local (foreign_levels)
display `"`foreign_levels'"'
foreach i of local foreign_levels{
local names: label origin `i'
preserve
qui keep if foreign == `i'
qui keep if _n == (_N - 1)
tempname weight
scalar `weight' = weight
restore
display "The second largest weight for category " `"`names'"' " was " %5.0fc `weight'
" kg"
}
```

```
. sysuse auto, clear
(1978 Automobile Data)

. sort foreign weight

. levelsof foreign, local (foreign_levels)
0 1

. display `"`foreign_levels'"'
0 1

. foreach i of local foreign_levels{
  2. local names: label origin `i'
  3. preserve
  4. qui keep if foreign == `i'
  5. qui keep if _n == (_N - 1)
  6. tempname weight
  7. scalar `weight' = weight
  8. restore
  9. display "The second largest weight for category " `"`names'"'
 10. display " was " %5.0fc `weight' " kg"
 11. }
The second largest weight for category Domestic
 was 4,720 kg
The second largest weight for category Foreign
 was 3,170 kg
```

VI. RECODE, XTILE AND CUT

a. Recode

Recode is usually used to create new categories for both categorical and/or continuous data.

Categorical data

In dataset auto, rep78, the variable can take values 1/5 inclusive as well as the value "missing". Assume you wish to recode this variable into three groups ("Low", "Medium" and "High") amalgamating the contents of levels 1&2, 3&4 and 5 into these new categories, respectively. You wish to create a new variable called new_rep78 and appropriate labels for the categorical variable.

```
sysuse auto, clear
recode rep78 (1/2 = 1 "Low") (3/4 = 2 "Medium") (5 = 3 "High") (missing = .), ///
pre(new_) label(new_rep78_label)
tabulate rep78 new_rep78
```

```
.
. sysuse auto, clear
(1978 Automobile Data)

. recode rep78 (1/2 = 1 "Low") (3/4 = 2 "Medium") (5 = 3 "High") (missing = .)
> pre(new_) label(new_rep78_label)
(67 differences between rep78 and new_rep78)

. tabulate rep78 new_rep78
```

Repair Record 1978	RECODE of rep78 (Repair Record 1978) Low	Medium	High	Total
1	2	0	0	2
2	8	0	0	8
3	0	30	0	30
4	0	18	0	18
5	0	0	11	11
Total	10	48	11	69

Continuous data

Examine the continuous variable mpg.

```
codebook mpg

------------------------------------------------------------------------------
mpg                                                             Mileage (mpg)
------------------------------------------------------------------------------

                  type:  numeric (int)

                 range:  [12,41]                      units:  1
         unique values:  21                       missing .:  0/74

                  mean:   21.2973
              std. dev:    5.7855

           percentiles:        10%       25%       50%       75%       90%
                                14        18        20        25        29
```

This variable is distributed between the values of 12 and 41 and appears to not be normally distributed. You could recode manually (e.g. min/20, 21/30, 31/40, 41/max), but some of the resulting categories may suffer from sparseness of data.

It's perhaps more logical to cut these data into quantiles.

b. xtile

Suppose, you wished to have the variable mpg cut into quintiles.

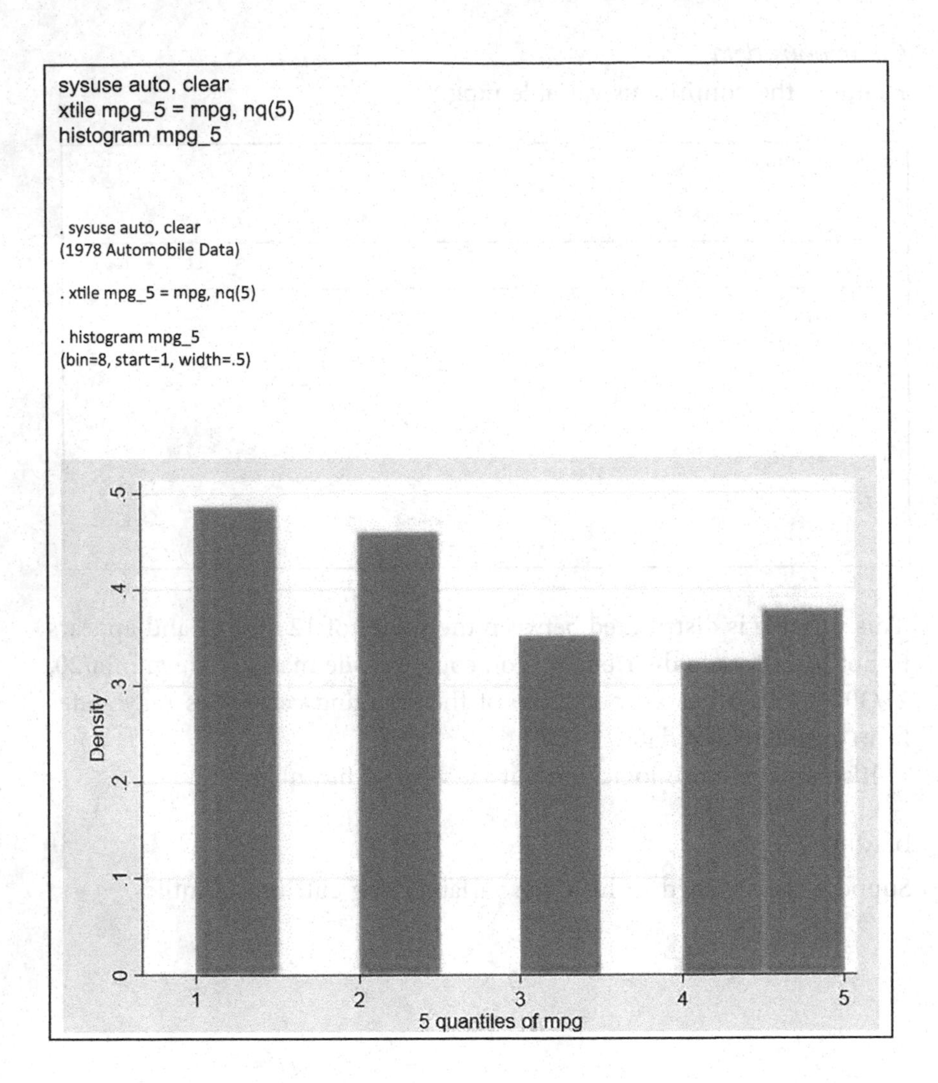
sysuse auto, clear
xtile mpg_5 = mpg, nq(5)
histogram mpg_5
. sysuse auto, clear
(1978 Automobile Data)
. xtile mpg_5 = mpg, nq(5)
. histogram mpg_5
(bin=8, start=1, width=.5)
Density
0
.1
.2
.3
.4
.5
1
2
3
4
5
5 quantiles of mpg

c. cut

An alternative would be to cut the variable into five equal-sized categories using egen cut. The options icodes and labels automatically produce labels starting from 0 at the lowest cut and indicate the positions of the cut in the labels themselves.

```
sysuse auto, clear
egen mpg_5 = cut (mpg), group(5) icodes label
histogram mpg_5
codebook mpg_5
```

```
. sysuse auto, clear
(1978 Automobile Data)

. egen mpg_5 = cut (mpg), group(5) icodes label

. histogram mpg_5
(bin=8, start=0, width=.5)

. codebook mpg_5

-------------------------------------------------------------------------------
mpg_5                                                               (unlabeled)
-------------------------------------------------------------------------------

                  type:  numeric (float)
                 label:  mpg_5

                 range:  [0,4]                        units:  1
         unique values:  5                        missing .:  0/74

            tabulation:  Freq.   Numeric  Label
                            14         0  12-
                            13         1  17-
                            16         2  19-
                            12         3  22-
                            19         4  25-
```

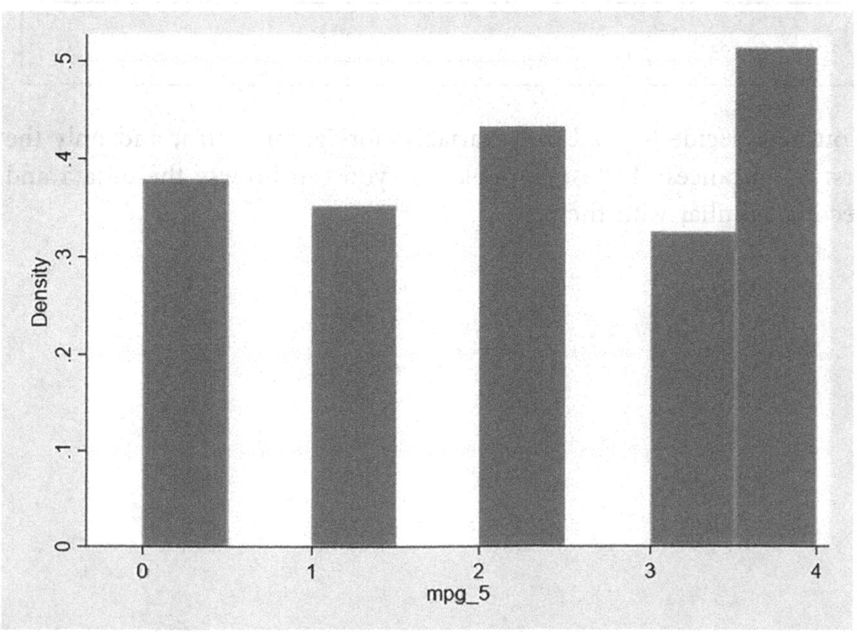

VII. USE AND USING

Some datasets are so large that they cannot be loaded into Stata at one go, or, they might take a very long time. You can list the variables in a dataset without loading it:

```
clear
describe using "`c(pwd)'/Data_In/Stata_Data/auto.dta"

. clear

. describe using "`c(pwd)'/Data_In/Stata_Data/auto.dta"

Contains data                                    1978 Automobile Data
  obs:            74                             21 Apr 2019 16:40
 vars:            12
 size:         3,478
--------------------------------------------------------------------------------
> -
               storage   display    value
variable name    type    format     label      variable label
--------------------------------------------------------------------------------
make            str18    %-18s                 Make and Model
price           int      %8.0gc                Price
mpg             int      %8.0g                 Mileage (mpg)
rep78           int      %8.0g                 Repair Record 1978
headroom        float    %6.1f                 Headroom (in.)
trunk           int      %8.0g                 Trunk space (cu. ft.)
weight          int      %8.0gc                Weight (lbs.)
length          int      %8.0g                 Length (in.)
turn            int      %8.0g                 Turn Circle (ft.)
displacement    int      %8.0g                 Displacement (cu. in.)
gear_ratio      float    %6.2f                 Gear Ratio
foreign         byte     %8.0g      origin     Car type
--------------------------------------------------------------------------------
> -
Sorted by: foreign
```

You now decide to load only variables foreign and turn, and only the first 20 instances of these variables, so you can browse these data and become familiar with them.

```
use foreign turn in 1/20 using "`c(pwd)'/Data_In/Stata_Data/auto.dta", clear
list in 1/20

. use foreign turn in 1/20 using "`c(pwd)'/Data_In/Stata_Data/auto.dta", clear
(1978 Automobile Data)

. list in 1/20

     +-----------------+
     | turn    foreign |
     |-----------------|
  1. |   40   Domestic |
  2. |   40   Domestic |
  3. |   35   Domestic |
  4. |   40   Domestic |
  5. |   43   Domestic |
     |-----------------|
  6. |   43   Domestic |
  7. |   34   Domestic |
  8. |   42   Domestic |
  9. |   43   Domestic |
 10. |   42   Domestic |
     |-----------------|
 11. |   44   Domestic |
 12. |   43   Domestic |
 13. |   45   Domestic |
 14. |   34   Domestic |
 15. |   43   Domestic |
     |-----------------|
 16. |   31   Domestic |
 17. |   41   Domestic |
 18. |   40   Domestic |
 19. |   43   Domestic |
 20. |   35   Domestic |
     +-----------------+
```

VII. MISSING VALUES

Stata stores missing values as very large numbers. If you receive a dataset where the missing values are recorded as any other value than ".", it is easier to just recode them to the default value of "." using the recode command. It is possible to identify different categories of missing values for Stata, but it's not worth the effort in most cases. The commands **misstable summarize** and **misstable patterns** can help to evaluate missingness in a dataset.

CHAPTER 10

Helpful Hints When Doing Regression

I. WHAT IS REGRESSION ANALYSIS?

The emphasis of this textbook is on coding and programming. However, the ultimate goal of programmers in the fields of statistics and data management is to analyse data and to produce results which further the research question. Regression and survival analyses are very commonly encountered statistical methods used in the analyses of real-world data. It is helpful to introduce these two statistical concepts, in particular, briefly here. A more exhaustive explanation of statistical concepts is beyond the scope of this textbook, and the reader should refer to more authoritative guides on these issues.

Linear Regression

Linear regression is one of several methods used in statistics to estimate the relationship between at least two variables (at least one of which is called the outcome (or dependent) and at least one of which is called the independent (or predictor) variable). The magnitude of the association, the precision of the estimate of the magnitude and the probability that the results could have been obtained by chance are almost always of interest in regression analyses. Stata uses a reasonably intuitive syntax in regression analyses, which is explained later in the chapter.

DOI: 10.1201/9781003483779-10

Survival Analysis (Time to Event Analysis)

Survival analyses acquired their name because they were often, in the past, used to analyse the time of survival in cancer trials. The methods developed in this area of medicine have become much more widely applied and are more generically termed “time to event”. The analysis estimates the instantaneous probability of an event occurring (the hazard), and the outcome is a dichotomous event (occurred or did not occur). Censoring is encountered (where information is not observed for a participant in a study) and is adjusted for in the analyses.

II. ENTERING CONTINUOUS AND CATEGORICAL VARIABLES

Categorical variables are entered with the prefix “i.” in front of the variable name, so Stata knows not to treat them as continuous variables. You need to do this even if you were to examine the variable using “codebook” and see that Stata has already figured out that the values are discrete.

Let’s use the auto dataset and regress a combination of continuous and discrete variables.

```
      Source |       SS           df       MS      Number of obs   =        74
-------------+----------------------------------   F(2, 71)        =      5.25
       Model |  81816017.5         2  40908008.7   Prob > F        =    0.0075
    Residual |   553249379        71  7792244.77   R-squared       =    0.1288
-------------+----------------------------------   Adj R-squared   =    0.1043
       Total |   635065396        73  8699525.97   Root MSE        =    2791.5

------------------------------------------------------------------------------
       price |      Coef.   Std. Err.      t    P>|t|     [95% Conf. Interval]
-------------+----------------------------------------------------------------
       trunk |   262.7717   81.85189     3.21   0.002     99.56364    425.9797
     foreign |   1190.155   760.8049     1.56   0.122    -326.8468    2707.157
       _cons |   2196.541   1267.857     1.73   0.088    -331.4939    4724.576
------------------------------------------------------------------------------
```

Since foreign is categorical and has only two values, the coefficient is correct, but unless you verify this elsewhere, you would not immediately know which value is being taken as the reference value. When you specify i.foreign, the label of the value appears.

```
sysuse auto,clear
regress price trunk i.foreign
```

```
. sysuse auto,clear
(1978 Automobile Data)

. regress price trunk i.foreign

      Source |       SS           df       MS      Number of obs   =        74
-------------+----------------------------------   F(2, 71)        =      5.25
       Model |  81816017.5         2  40908008.7   Prob > F        =    0.0075
    Residual |   553249379        71  7792244.77   R-squared       =    0.1288
-------------+----------------------------------   Adj R-squared   =    0.1043
       Total |   635065396        73  8699525.97   Root MSE        =    2791.5

------------------------------------------------------------------------------
       price |      Coef.   Std. Err.      t    P>|t|     [95% Conf. Interval]
-------------+----------------------------------------------------------------
       trunk |   262.7717   81.85189     3.21   0.002     99.56364    425.9797
             |
     foreign |
     Foreign |   1190.155   760.8049     1.56   0.122    -326.8468    2707.157
       _cons |   2196.541   1267.857     1.73   0.088    -331.4939    4724.576
------------------------------------------------------------------------------
```

The variable "rep78" has more than two values and is categorical. Let's use this variable in a similar regression and observe the results.

```
sysuse auto, clear
regress price trunk i.rep78
```

```
. sysuse auto, clear
(1978 Automobile Data)

. regress price trunk i.rep78

      Source |       SS           df       MS      Number of obs   =        69
-------------+----------------------------------   F(5, 63)        =      1.53
       Model |  62501990.5         5  12500398.1   Prob > F        =    0.1929
    Residual |   514294968        63   8163412.2   R-squared       =    0.1084
-------------+----------------------------------   Adj R-squared   =    0.0376
       Total |   576796959        68  8482308.22   Root MSE        =    2857.2

------------------------------------------------------------------------------
       price |      Coef.   Std. Err.      t    P>|t|     [95% Conf. Interval]
-------------+----------------------------------------------------------------
       trunk |    222.313   86.32485     2.58   0.012     49.80657    394.8195
             |
       rep78 |
          2  |   41.45775   2319.849     0.02   0.986     -4594.39    4677.306
          3  |   360.4152   2166.802     0.17   0.868    -3969.592    4690.423
          4  |   395.4349   2172.908     0.18   0.856    -3946.775    4737.645
          5  |   691.6661   2211.082     0.31   0.755     -3726.83    5110.162
             |
       _cons |   2674.839   2149.444     1.24   0.218    -1620.483    6970.161
------------------------------------------------------------------------------
```

III. CHANGING THE REFERENCE VALUE

You can infer that Stata has chosen the value "1" to be the baseline value for comparison as it is not listed in the output. This may not be convenient. Stata automatically chooses the lowest value for comparison. However, if you are, for example, using BMI as a variable, the lowest values correspond to "underweight", and you would prefer to choose "normal weight" as the comparator value. You can specify which value you wish to make the baseline by indicating the value to Stata as below. In this case, we choose the value "2" to be the reference value.

```
sysuse auto, clear
regress price trunk ib2.rep78
```

```
. sysuse auto, clear
(1978 Automobile Data)

. regress price trunk ib2.rep78

      Source |       SS           df       MS      Number of obs   =        69
-------------+----------------------------------   F(5, 63)        =      1.53
       Model |  62501990.5         5  12500398.1   Prob > F        =    0.1929
    Residual |   514294968        63   8163412.2   R-squared       =    0.1084
-------------+----------------------------------   Adj R-squared   =    0.0376
       Total |   576796959        68  8482308.22   Root MSE        =    2857.2

------------------------------------------------------------------------------
       price |      Coef.   Std. Err.      t    P>|t|     [95% Conf. Interval]
-------------+----------------------------------------------------------------
       trunk |    222.313   86.32485     2.58   0.012     49.80657    394.8195
             |
       rep78 |
          1  |  -41.45775   2319.849    -0.02   0.986    -4677.306     4594.39
          3  |   318.9575   1138.248     0.28   0.780     -1955.65    2593.565
          4  |   353.9771   1217.941     0.29   0.772    -2079.884    2787.838
          5  |   650.2083    1355.53     0.48   0.633    -2058.601    3359.018
             |
       _cons |   2716.297   1616.891     1.68   0.098    -514.8009    5947.395
------------------------------------------------------------------------------
```

The output now omits value "2" for rep78 as this is now the reference value.

IV. INTERACTION TERMS

Let's repeat the regression above but include an interaction term between rep78 and foreign.

```
sysuse auto, clear
regress price trunk ib2.rep78 ib2.rep78#i.foreign
```

```
. sysuse auto, clear
(1978 Automobile Data)

. regress price trunk ib2.rep78 ib2.rep78#i.foreign
note: 1.rep78#1.foreign identifies no observations in the sample
note: 2b.rep78#1.foreign identifies no observations in the sample

      Source |       SS           df       MS      Number of obs   =        69
-------------+----------------------------------   F(8, 60)        =      1.30
       Model |  85296763.3         8  10662095.4   Prob > F        =    0.2602
    Residual |   491500196        60  8191669.93   R-squared       =    0.1479
-------------+----------------------------------   Adj R-squared   =    0.0343
       Total |   576796959        68  8482308.22   Root MSE        =    2862.1

------------------------------------------------------------------------------
       price |      Coef.   Std. Err.      t    P>|t|     [95% Conf. Interval]
-------------+----------------------------------------------------------------
       trunk |   262.9013   96.64937     2.72   0.009     69.57374    456.2288
             |
       rep78 |
          1  |   207.1453   2338.852     0.09   0.930    -4471.256    4885.547
          3  |   385.0678   1155.898     0.33   0.740    -1927.072    2697.207
          4  |  -622.8262   1404.664    -0.44   0.659    -3432.573    2186.921
          5  |   -415.756   2316.278    -0.18   0.858    -5049.002     4217.49
             |
rep78#foreign |
   1#Foreign |          0  (empty)
   2#Foreign |          0  (empty)
   3#Foreign |   -921.544   1770.079    -0.52   0.605    -4462.229    2619.141
   4#Foreign |    2044.93   1481.571     1.38   0.173    -918.6533    5008.514
   5#Foreign |   1460.125   2249.295     0.65   0.519    -3039.135    5959.385
             |
       _cons |   2122.694   1738.371     1.22   0.227    -1354.565    5599.953
------------------------------------------------------------------------------
```

However, if you wish the coefficients of regression for both of the interaction terms plus the coefficients of the interactions themselves, then issue the command with two hash signs as below:

```
sysuse auto, clear
regress price trunk ib2.rep78##i.foreign
```

```
.
. sysuse auto, clear
(1978 Automobile Data)

. regress price trunk ib2.rep78##i.foreign
note: 1.rep78#1.foreign identifies no observations in the sample
note: 2b.rep78#1.foreign identifies no observations in the sample
note: 5.rep78#1.foreign omitted because of collinearity

      Source |       SS           df       MS      Number of obs   =        69
-------------+----------------------------------   F(8, 60)        =      1.30
       Model |  85296763.3         8  10662095.4   Prob > F        =    0.2602
    Residual |   491500196        60  8191669.93   R-squared       =    0.1479
-------------+----------------------------------   Adj R-squared   =    0.0343
       Total |   576796959        68  8482308.22   Root MSE        =    2862.1

------------------------------------------------------------------------------
       price |      Coef.   Std. Err.      t    P>|t|     [95% Conf. Interval]
-------------+----------------------------------------------------------------
       trunk |   262.9013   96.64937     2.72   0.009     69.57374    456.2288
             |
       rep78 |
          1  |   207.1453   2338.852     0.09   0.930    -4471.256    4885.547
          3  |   385.0678   1155.898     0.33   0.740    -1927.072    2697.207
          4  |  -622.8262   1404.664    -0.44   0.659    -3432.573    2186.921
          5  |   -415.756   2316.278    -0.18   0.858    -5049.002     4217.49
             |
     foreign |
    Foreign  |   1460.125   2249.295     0.65   0.519    -3039.135    5959.385
             |
rep78#foreign|
  1#Foreign  |          0  (empty)
  2#Foreign  |          0  (empty)
  3#Foreign  |  -2381.669   2887.554    -0.82   0.413    -8157.637    3394.299
  4#Foreign  |   584.8055   2745.366     0.21   0.832    -4906.745    6076.356
  5#Foreign  |          0  (omitted)
             |
       _cons |   2122.694   1738.371     1.22   0.227    -1354.565    5599.953
------------------------------------------------------------------------------
```

You can include a continuous variable in an interaction term.

```
sysuse auto, clear
regress price trunk ib2.rep78##c.weight
```

```
. do "C:\Users\rmjlasg\AppData\Local\Temp\STD3590_000000.tmp"

. sysuse auto, clear
(1978 Automobile Data)

. regress price trunk ib2.rep78##c.weight

      Source |       SS           df       MS      Number of obs   =        69
-------------+----------------------------------   F(10, 58)       =      6.52
       Model |  305240464        10  30524046.4   Prob > F        =    0.0000
    Residual |  271556495        58  4682008.53   R-squared       =    0.5292
-------------+----------------------------------   Adj R-squared   =    0.4480
       Total |  576796959        68  8482308.22   Root MSE        =    2163.8

------------------------------------------------------------------------------
       price |      Coef.   Std. Err.      t    P>|t|     [95% Conf. Interval]
-------------+----------------------------------------------------------------
       trunk |  -93.02845   92.63588    -1.00   0.319    -278.4593    92.40241
             |
       rep78 |
          1  |    16168.2   14786.59     1.09   0.279    -13430.38    45766.77
          3  |   8332.695   6854.557     1.22   0.229    -5388.192    22053.58
          4  |   17117.77   6689.207     2.56   0.013     3727.869    30507.68
          5  |   5822.812   7626.413     0.76   0.448    -9443.113    21088.74
             |
      weight |   5.983687   2.051667     2.92   0.005     1.876829    10.09054
             |
rep78#c.weight |
          1  |  -5.362181   4.705491    -1.14   0.259    -14.78124    4.056882
          3  |  -2.268501    2.02263    -1.12   0.267    -6.317236    1.780233
          4  |  -4.956079   1.990932    -2.49   0.016    -8.941363   -.9707946
          5  |  -.0013182   2.553213    -0.00   1.000     -5.11213    5.109493
             |
       _cons |  -12739.62   6434.572    -1.98   0.052    -25619.82    140.5717
------------------------------------------------------------------------------
```

V. OMITTING LEVELS FROM THE REGRESSION

Run the regression, but this time omit level 4 of rep78 while using level 2 as the baseline. You will need to omit the interaction term (which if present will force Stata to display all the coefficients for rep78 except the baseline).

```
sysuse auto, clear
regress price trunk ib2o4.rep78 i.foreign
```

```
. sysuse auto, clear
(1978 Automobile Data)

. regress price trunk ib2o4.rep78 i.foreign

      Source |       SS           df       MS      Number of obs   =        69
-------------+----------------------------------   F(5, 63)        =      1.74
       Model |  70124912.1         5  14024982.4   Prob > F        =    0.1376
    Residual |   506672047        63  8042413.44   R-squared       =    0.1216
-------------+----------------------------------   Adj R-squared   =    0.0519
       Total |   576796959        68  8482308.22   Root MSE        =    2835.9

------------------------------------------------------------------------------
       price |      Coef.   Std. Err.      t    P>|t|     [95% Conf. Interval]
-------------+----------------------------------------------------------------
       trunk |   252.1141   90.95785     2.77   0.007      70.3493    433.8788
             |
       rep78 |
          1  |   205.2474   2187.074     0.09   0.926    -4165.271    4575.766
          3  |   267.9692   792.1523     0.34   0.736    -1315.021    1850.959
          4  |          0  (omitted)
          5  |   23.08511   1104.487     0.02   0.983    -2184.056    2230.226
             |
     foreign |
     Foreign |   960.3976   944.6676     1.02   0.313      -927.37    2848.165
       _cons |   2216.283   1511.834     1.47   0.148    -804.8758    5237.442
------------------------------------------------------------------------------
```

VI. DISPLAYING COEFFICIENTS FOR ONLY GIVEN LEVELS

To display only the coefficient for level 2 of rep78 in the regression, use the following code:

```
sysuse auto, clear
regress price trunk 2.rep78 i.foreign
```

```
. sysuse auto, clear
(1978 Automobile Data)

. regress price trunk 2.rep78 i.foreign

      Source |       SS           df       MS      Number of obs   =        69
-------------+----------------------------------   F(3, 65)        =      2.96
       Model |  69252012.4         3  23084004.1   Prob > F        =    0.0388
    Residual |   507544947        65  7808383.79   R-squared       =    0.1201
-------------+----------------------------------   Adj R-squared   =    0.0795
       Total |   576796959        68  8482308.22   Root MSE        =    2794.3

------------------------------------------------------------------------------
       price |      Coef.   Std. Err.      t    P>|t|     [95% Conf. Interval]
-------------+----------------------------------------------------------------
       trunk |   253.3003   85.42829     2.97   0.004     82.68817    423.9123
     2.rep78 |  -114.6349   1083.266    -0.11   0.916    -2278.066    2048.797
             |
     foreign |
     Foreign |   833.7249   823.0618     1.01   0.315    -810.0431    2477.493
       _cons |   2377.744   1369.597     1.74   0.087    -357.5306    5113.018
------------------------------------------------------------------------------
```

VII. TO USE THE CATEGORY WITH THE HIGHEST FREQUENCY OF VALUES AS THE REFERENCE LEVEL

The value 3 of the variable rep78 contains the greatest number of items (n = 30). The prefix ib(freq) will identify to Stata that the level with the largest number of observations should be used as the baseline. An example is given below.

```
sysuse auto, clear
codebook rep78
```

```
.
. sysuse auto, clear
(1978 Automobile Data)

. codebook rep78

-------------------------------------------------------------------------------
rep78                                                        Repair Record 1978
-------------------------------------------------------------------------------

                  type:  numeric (int)

                 range:  [1,5]                        units:  1
         unique values:  5                        missing .:  5/74

            tabulation:  Freq.  Value
                             2  1
                             8  2
                            30  3
                            18  4
                            11  5
                             5  .
```

VIII. USING NO REFERENCE CATEGORY

It is possible to have Stata display all the levels for a variable in a regression.

In this example, both levels of foreign should be displayed.

```
sysuse auto, clear
regress price trunk rep78 ibn.foreign
```

```
. sysuse auto, clear
(1978 Automobile Data)

. regress price trunk rep78 ibn.foreign
note: 1.foreign omitted because of collinearity

      Source |       SS           df       MS      Number of obs   =        69
-------------+----------------------------------   F(3, 65)        =      2.96
       Model |  69353253.8         3  23117751.3   Prob > F        =    0.0386
    Residual |   507443705        65  7806826.23   R-squared       =    0.1202
-------------+----------------------------------   Adj R-squared   =    0.0796
       Total |   576796959        68  8482308.22   Root MSE        =    2794.1

------------------------------------------------------------------------------
       price |      Coef.   Std. Err.      t    P>|t|     [95% Conf. Interval]
-------------+----------------------------------------------------------------
       trunk |   255.1929   85.88346     2.97   0.004     83.67177     426.714
       rep78 |  -66.45997   427.4935    -0.16   0.877    -920.2235    787.3036
             |
     foreign |
    Domestic |  -944.0822   986.3055    -0.96   0.342     -2913.87    1025.706
     Foreign |          0  (omitted)
             |
       _cons |   3474.937   2066.088     1.68   0.097    -651.3249    7601.199
------------------------------------------------------------------------------
```

Note that one level of foreign has been dropped because of collinearity.

IX. USING THE LAST LEVEL OF A CATEGORICAL VARIABLE AS REFERENCE

```
sysuse auto, clear
regress price trunk ib(last).rep78 i.foreign
```

```
. sysuse auto, clear
(1978 Automobile Data)

. regress price trunk ib(last).rep78 i.foreign

      Source |       SS           df       MS      Number of obs   =        69
-------------+----------------------------------   F(6, 62)        =      1.43
       Model |  70180116.9         6  11696686.1   Prob > F        =    0.2171
    Residual |   506616842        62  8171239.39   R-squared       =    0.1217
-------------+----------------------------------   Adj R-squared   =    0.0367
       Total |   576796959        68  8482308.22   Root MSE        =    2858.5

------------------------------------------------------------------------------
       price |      Coef.   Std. Err.      t    P>|t|     [95% Conf. Interval]
-------------+----------------------------------------------------------------
       trunk |   252.5189   91.81568     2.75   0.008     68.98201    436.0559
             |
       rep78 |
           1 |   208.3783     2399.1     0.09   0.931    -4587.353     5004.11
           2 |    64.8249   1543.804     0.04   0.967    -3021.195    3150.845
           3 |   265.3025   1225.701     0.22   0.829     -2184.84    2715.445
           4 |    -42.705     1138.6    -0.04   0.970    -2318.733    2233.323
             |
     foreign |
     Foreign |   990.9774   1022.304     0.97   0.336    -1052.579    3034.534
       _cons |   2209.711   1773.596     1.25   0.217    -1335.657    5755.078
------------------------------------------------------------------------------
```

X. DISPLAYING THE BASELINE LEVEL

```
sysuse auto, clear
regress price trunk ib(freq).rep78 i.foreign, baselevels
```

```
.
. sysuse auto, clear
(1978 Automobile Data)

. regress price trunk ib(freq).rep78 i.foreign, baselevels

      Source |       SS           df       MS      Number of obs   =        69
-------------+----------------------------------   F(6, 62)        =      1.43
       Model |  70180116.9         6  11696686.1   Prob > F        =    0.2171
    Residual |   506616842        62  8171239.39   R-squared       =    0.1217
-------------+----------------------------------   Adj R-squared   =    0.0367
       Total |   576796959        68  8482308.22   Root MSE        =    2858.5

------------------------------------------------------------------------------
       price |      Coef.   Std. Err.      t    P>|t|     [95% Conf. Interval]
-------------+----------------------------------------------------------------
       trunk |   252.5189   91.81568     2.75   0.008     68.98201    436.0559
             |
       rep78 |
          1  |  -56.92417   2190.332    -0.03   0.979    -4435.335    4321.487
          2  |  -200.4776   1145.334    -0.18   0.862    -2489.967    2089.012
          3  |          0  (base)
          4  |  -308.0075   935.3276    -0.33   0.743    -2177.701    1561.686
          5  |  -265.3025   1225.701    -0.22   0.829    -2715.445     2184.84
             |
     foreign |
   Domestic  |          0  (base)
    Foreign  |   990.9774   1022.304     0.97   0.336    -1052.579    3034.534
             |
       _cons |   2475.013    1531.31     1.62   0.111    -586.0311    5536.058
------------------------------------------------------------------------------
```

XI. SPECIFYING LEVELS TO BE USED IN THE REGRESSION USING ONLY LEVELS 3 AND 4 OF REP78

```
sysuse auto, clear
regress price trunk i(3,4).rep78 i.foreign, baselevels
```

```
. sysuse auto, clear
(1978 Automobile Data)

. regress price trunk i(3,4).rep78 i.foreign, baselevels

      Source |       SS           df       MS      Number of obs   =        69
-------------+----------------------------------   F(3, 65)        =      2.97
       Model |  69627424.8         3  23209141.6   Prob > F        =    0.0380
    Residual |   507169534        65  7802608.22   R-squared       =    0.1207
-------------+----------------------------------   Adj R-squared   =    0.0801
       Total |   576796959        68  8482308.22   Root MSE        =    2793.3

------------------------------------------------------------------------------
       price |      Coef.   Std. Err.      t    P>|t|     [95% Conf. Interval]
-------------+----------------------------------------------------------------
       trunk |   254.7148   85.41954     2.98   0.004      84.1202    425.3094
             |
       rep78 |
          3  |          0  (base)
          4  |  -193.0055   792.4409    -0.24   0.808    -1775.619    1389.608
             |
     foreign |
    Domestic |          0  (base)
    Foreign  |   904.7307   825.7856     1.10   0.277    -744.4769    2553.938
             |
       _cons |    2373.49   1351.229     1.76   0.084    -325.0999     5072.08
------------------------------------------------------------------------------
```

Using levels 3 and 4 of rep78 and specifying that level 4 be used as the baseline and with no constant in the regression:

```
sysuse auto,clear
regress price trunk i(3,4)b4.rep78 i.foreign, baselevels noconstant
```

```
. sysuse auto,clear
(1978 Automobile Data)

. regress price trunk i(3,4)b4.rep78 i.foreign, baselevels noconstant

      Source |       SS           df       MS      Number of obs   =        69
-------------+----------------------------------   F(3, 66)        =    110.59
       Model |  2.6550e+09         3   885000953   Prob > F        =    0.0000
    Residual |   528189779        66  8002875.44   R-squared       =    0.8341
-------------+----------------------------------   Adj R-squared   =    0.8265
       Total |  3.1832e+09        69  46133226.7   Root MSE        =    2828.9

------------------------------------------------------------------------------
       price |      Coef.   Std. Err.      t    P>|t|     [95% Conf. Interval]
-------------+----------------------------------------------------------------
       trunk |   379.1766   36.80215    10.30   0.000     305.6988    452.6545
             |
       rep78 |
          3  |   468.0707    741.119     0.63   0.530    -1011.621    1947.763
          4  |          0  (base)
             |
     foreign |
   Domestic  |          0  (base)
    Foreign  |   1723.997   708.6363     2.43   0.018     309.1587    3138.835
------------------------------------------------------------------------------
```

XII. SPECIFYING BASELINE LEVEL AS SECOND LEVEL OF A VARIABLE

```
sysuse auto, clear
codebook rep78
regress price trunk ib(#2).rep78 i.foreign, baselevels
```

```
. sysuse auto, clear
(1978 Automobile Data)

. codebook rep78

------------------------------------------------------------------------------
rep78                                                       Repair Record 1978
------------------------------------------------------------------------------

                  type:  numeric (int)

                 range:  [1,5]                        units:  1
         unique values:  5                        missing .:  5/74

            tabulation:  Freq.  Value
                             2  1
                             8  2
                            30  3
                            18  4
                            11  5
                             5  .

. regress price trunk ib(#2).rep78 i.foreign, baselevels

      Source |       SS           df       MS      Number of obs   =        69
-------------+----------------------------------   F(6, 62)        =      1.43
       Model |  70180116.9         6  11696686.1   Prob > F        =    0.2171
    Residual |   506616842        62  8171239.39   R-squared       =    0.1217
-------------+----------------------------------   Adj R-squared   =    0.0367
       Total |   576796959        68  8482308.22   Root MSE        =    2858.5

------------------------------------------------------------------------------
       price |      Coef.   Std. Err.      t    P>|t|     [95% Conf. Interval]
-------------+----------------------------------------------------------------
       trunk |   252.5189   91.81568     2.75   0.008     68.98201    436.0559
             |
       rep78 |
          1  |   143.5534   2328.795     0.06   0.951    -4511.641    4798.748
          2  |          0  (base)
          3  |   200.4776   1145.334     0.18   0.862    -2089.012    2489.967
          4  |  -107.5299   1308.232    -0.08   0.935    -2722.648    2507.588
          5  |   -64.8249   1543.804    -0.04   0.967    -3150.845    3021.195
             |
     foreign |
    Domestic |          0  (base)
     Foreign |   990.9774   1022.304     0.97   0.336    -1052.579    3034.534
             |
       _cons |   2274.536   1680.633     1.35   0.181    -1085.002    5634.074
------------------------------------------------------------------------------
```

CHAPTER 11

Time Series Operators and Survival Analyses

I. TIME SERIES OPERATORS

Load the dataset entitled "gym". It contains serial measurements of weights for individuals. Stata refers to this type of data as "panel" data. In the United Kingdom, this type of data often referred to as longitudinal cohort data. Most frequently, lags, leads, differences and seasonal differences of a variable are investigated.

use https://www.stata-press.com/data/r18/gymdata

```
use "`c(pwd)'/Data_In/Stata_Data/gym.dta", clear

. use "`c(pwd)'/Data_In/Stata_Data/gym.dta", clear
```

For time series analyses, it is necessary for Stata to identify the id and time variables (in that order) using the command **xtset.**

```
xtset id month

. xtset id month
       panel variable:  id (unbalanced)
        time variable:  month, 1 to 12, but with gaps
                delta:  1 unit
```

DOI: 10.1201/9781003483779-11

Note the Stata display which indicates the difference between time units (delta), the id variable and whether or not the data contain gaps.

II. SURVIVAL ANALYSES

Survival data are also longitudinal cohort data with a variable that indicates if an event has been reached or if the individual has been "censored". Definitions of these terms are beyond this manual but revise survival analysis if necessary. Load the dataset that contains data about time to death for patients with cancer.

```
webuse cancer, clear

(Patient Survival in Drug Trial)
```

To analyse these data, it is necessary to "stset" the data – i.e. to indicate to Stata that these data are about time to events. The first variable that must be specified is the time variable in the study. The option then includes the failure variable (1 is usually used to code that the outcome of interest has occurred).

```
stset studytime

. stset studytime

     failure event:  (assumed to fail at time=studytime)
obs. time interval:  (0, studytime]
 exit on or before:  failure

------------------------------------------------------------------------------
         48  total observations
          0  exclusions
------------------------------------------------------------------------------
         48  observations remaining, representing
         48  failures in single-record/single-failure data
        744  total analysis time at risk and under observation
                                                at risk from t =         0
                                     earliest observed entry t =         0
                                          last observed exit t =        39
```

Stata has created four new variables.

_t0 indicates if the event has occurred before time 0. This column should usually contains only 0's; otherwise, there may be an error in your data. _t is the time since analysis has begun (the origin). _d is whether or not the event has occurred. _st indicates whether or not the observation row for that individual is being used in the analyses.

To graph the survival curve with 95% confidence intervals:

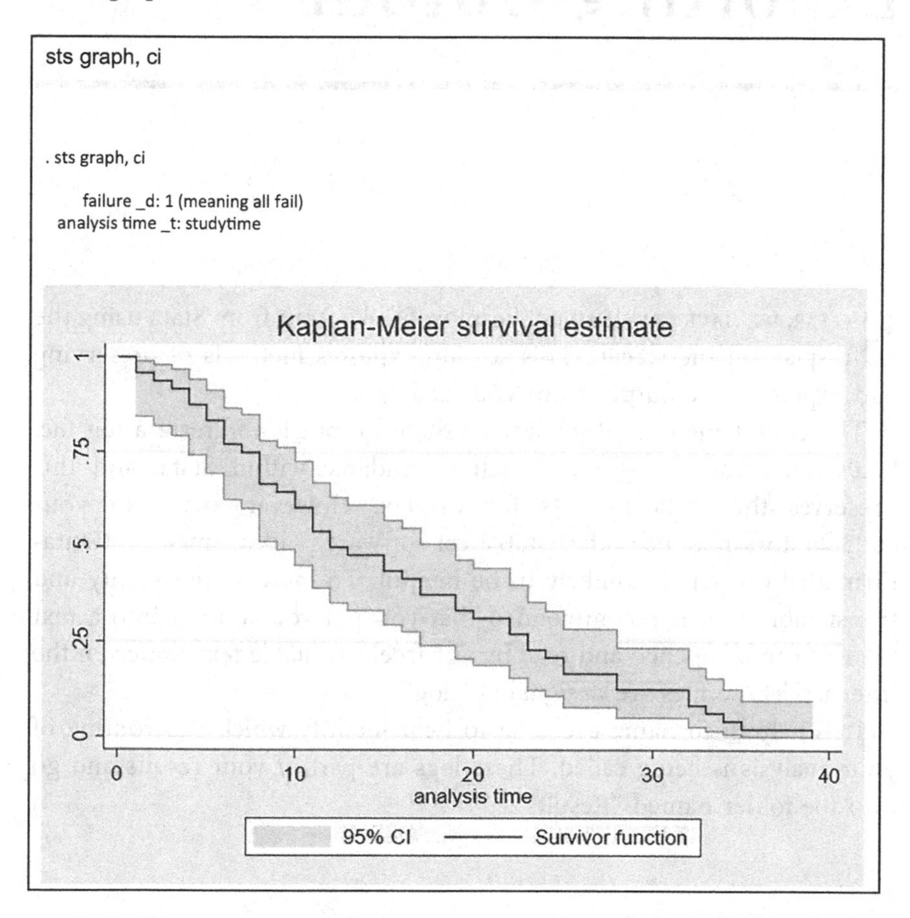

To remove the stset variables:

```
stset, clear

stset, clear
```

CHAPTER 12

Exporting Output

SO FAR, WE HAVE EXAMINED THE results of the output from Stata using the display on the screen. This section explores methods of preserving and exploring the output from your analyses.

The easiest method of preserving Stata output is to create a log file. Stata can create a log file, which is readable within Stata, and this preserves the Stata formats for display. However, many of your collaborators may use other statistical software, and a .smcl file (Stata-formatted output) is unlikely to be helpful. To increase portability and transferability, it is recommended that you put your output into a text file that can be opened and read by any freely available text reader on the internet. These files are designated ".log".

It is helpful to name each log to help identify which sub-routine of your analysis is being called. These logs are part of your results and go into the folder named "Results".

DOI: 10.1201/9781003483779-12

```
log using "`c(pwd)'/Results/Routine_1.log", replace name ("Routine_1")

sysuse auto, clear
regress weight price i.foreign

log close Routine_1
```

```
. log using "`c(pwd)'/Results/Routine_1.log", replace name ("Routine_1")
--------------------------------------------------------------------------------
      name:  Routine_1
       log:
  c:\Analysis_Folder/Results/Routine_1.log log
  type:  text

. sysuse auto, clear
(1978 Automobile Data)

. regress weight price i.foreign

      Source |       SS           df       MS      Number of obs   =        74
-------------+----------------------------------   F(2, 71)        =     73.48
       Model |    29731062         2    14865531   Prob > F        =    0.0000
    Residual |  14363116.4        71  202297.414   R-squared       =    0.6743
-------------+----------------------------------   Adj R-squared   =    0.6651
       Total |  44094178.4        73  604029.841   Root MSE        =    449.77

------------------------------------------------------------------------------
      weight |      Coef.   Std. Err.      t    P>|t|     [95% Conf. Interval]
-------------+----------------------------------------------------------------
       price |   .1498907   .0178691     8.39   0.000     .1142608    .1855206
             |
     foreign |
     Foreign |  -1048.011   114.5286    -9.15   0.000    -1276.375   -819.6474
       _cons |   2406.916   125.1577    19.23   0.000     2157.359    2656.473
------------------------------------------------------------------------------

.
. log close Routine_1
      name:  Routine_1
       log:  c:\EHR_Course/Results/Routine_1.log
  log type:  text
```

CHAPTER 13

Stata Programming

I. INTRODUCTION

A Stata program is simply a list of commands that the package executes in sequence. It is analogous to typing a series of commands, such as codebook, generate and describe, for example, and Stata executing them in sequence.

The extension .ado means "automatically executed do files. These files live in special folders (depending on where you get them from), and Stata automatically looks into these folders and will retrieve and run any program placed there.

II. .ADO FILE REPOSITORIES

To find the location of the Stata repositories, issue the command "sysdir" to Stata, and a list of directories appears in the output window.

```
. sysdir
   STATA:  C:\Program Files\Stata18\
    BASE:  C:\Program Files\Stata18\ado\base\
    SITE:  C:\Program Files\Stata18\ado\site\
    PLUS:  C:\ado\plus\
PERSONAL:  C:\ado\personal\
OLDPLACE:  C:\ado\
```


DOI: 10.1201/9781003483779-13

The sysdir command will show the relationship between the folder location and the name assigned by Stata. There are six original folders, although you can add to this sequence if you wish. It's never a good idea to change these filepaths, as Stata can stop working properly if it can't find where the programs it needs are located. However, the damage is only temporary. Simply restart Stata, and the default locations are restored.

STATA is the default location where the Stata program is located, and it is installed by default into the folder named "Program Files" in Windows.

BASE is where the original official .ado files are located that were downloaded with the Stata package when it was released. Any .ado files that have been updated in subsequent versions are also placed here.

PLUS is where packages that you download from the web are installed. To find user-written packages, use the command "search" to find .ado files that have been written by the Stata user community. "search" will search the Stata Journal, SSC Archives from Boston College (including programs from Statalist) and other locations on the web. Issuing the command "help net_mnu" will allow you to search the files associated with installation and maintenance of Stata using the Stata Journal, Stata Technical Bulletin and other community-contributed websites. As an exercise, download a package named "pretty_suite" which makes pretty baseline tables and tables of regression outputs easily. We will be reviewing this command later in the book when automated reporting is discussed. To do this, type *search pretty_suitee* in Stata, and the following screen appears:

```
search for pretty_suite

Search of official help files, FAQs, Examples, and Stata Journals

Search of web resources from Stata and other users

(contacting http://www.stata.com)

1 package found (Stata Journal listed first)
-----------------------------------------

pretty_suite from http://fmwww.bc.edu/RePEc/bocode/p
    'PRETTY_SUITE': module with programs to aid with routine reporting for
    clinical trials / pretty_suite contains a suite of programmes which are
    designed / to aid with routine reporting for clinical trials. The suite /
    comprised the programme pretty_baseline which makes routinely /

(click here to return to the previous screen)

(end of search)
```

FIGURE 13.1

Simply click on the http link at the top and then install the package from the subsequent screen.

An easier alternative is simply to issue the following command: "ssc install pretty_suite". The package is automatically installed in the PLUS folder. Check that the package and the associated help file are located in the folder. To remove the files, simply type ssc uninstall pretty_suite, for example.

To update user-written packages that are installed in the PLUS directory, issue the command *ado update, update.* If you do not issue the subcommand update, then a list of packages for which updates are available will be returned, but they will not be automatically installed. The command "help ado update" provides comprehensive information.

SITE is the location where your organisation may place commonly used files so that there is uniformity across all staff on a project, for example.

You can find where your PERSONAL directory is located by using the command "personal". The PERSONAL directory is where you copy the .ado files that you have written and that you have not submitted to one of the directories on the web that we have discussed above.

OLDPLACE is a very old .ado storage location and is not used anymore. It is very unlikely that you will ever need to access this folder. It is included for backward compatibility and was used in very early Stata versions.

You can, if you wish, add additional folders to those that are listed above. You do this by typing "adopath +" followed by the path you wish to add. Stata will then add this location to the end of the current directory pathway.

You can change the default location of any of the folders given above using the command "sysdir set" followed by the name of the folder type you wish to set (for example, PERSONAL or PLUS) and then followed by the filepath.

III. CREATING YOUR FIRST PROGRAM

The initial instruction "program" identifies the subsequent code as being a Stata program. This identifier is then followed by the name of the program. The end of the program is identified with the command "end" on a new line.

The program name that you assign cannot replicate any already existing Stata program name. The program instructions are placed between the introductory "program programname" and "end".

Once the program has been created and run for the first time, you can execute it by simply calling the program name you used in its creation in the first place.

It is inevitable that you will start by writing a program and then testing it in the real environment. As time goes on, you will likely fix bugs and increase the complexity of the program. However, once a program is defined and is run once, it is then stored in Stata's memory until the program exits. So, any attempt to fix the program in the .do file and re-run will end in failure as Stata will identify that the program already exists.

Therefore, it is common practice to prefix all programs with the following line of code which is displayed in the code snipped below. Let's assume you wish to amend the program named "pretty_baseline" that was downloaded earlier. You would find the file in the PLUS folder (having previously identified the location of the folders with "sysdir"), open it using a simple text package and paste the contents into a .do file of an active instance of Stata. If you attempt to access a .ado file by clicking on it, Stata will attempt to open the file and it will fail. You can only run the file by issuing a command within Stata, or you can open the file with a text application and copy it into a .do file. Or, you could locate and open the file using the inbuilt .do file editor in Stata.

IV. HELLO WORLD

Let's create a program that returns the greeting "Hello World" when you type the instruction "greeting" into an active Stata command window.

```
capture program drop greeting
program greeting
display "Hello World"
end
```

The instruction "capture" instructs Stata to ignore any errors that may arise from the first line. This can occur if you are running the instruction to drop the program for the first time, but the named program does not already exist. Then Stata will throw an error that the program does not exist. However, if you then remove the line and run the program more than once, Stata will throw the error that the program already exists on the second attempt to define the program!!

Once you have defined the program adequately and you are sure that it's running properly, you may wish to save this program and to have it loaded into Stata's programming environment every time you open Stata. One way would be to find the .do file where you created the program and to run it every time you opened Stata and then the program would be defined and loaded into Stata's memory.

Another more time-efficient method would be to save the file as an .ado file. This is done by accessing the file menu of the .do file window, and then selecting file type .ado from the "save as" submenu. Then place the files in the PERSONAL folder and every time Stata is opened, it will read the .ado file and your program will be loaded. You can then access the new program as you would any other Stata program.

V. STORED RESULTS

The results from programs can be stored in a variety of ways. This is important if you use your program to return results that you will use subsequently. We will now take a brief, but necessary, detour into reviewing how Stata saves stored results.

Stata commands are classified as being:

e-class estimation commands store results in e() – used to store results from estimation commands (e.g. regression modelling).

r-class commands store results in r() – used to store results from descriptive statistics commands (e.g. tabulate and summarize).

s-class parsing commands store results in s() – used in commands that parse and are not covered in this book.

n-class commands store output that is not stored in r(), e() or s(). This type of class is very rarely encountered.

c-class holds the values of system parameters and settings, along with some constants, such as the value of *e*.

The most commonly used commands producing statistical results store output in either r or e classes.

Commands that are used in simulations are usually either r or e class. Since this proposed program does not involve estimation, the appropriate class to return results is r class.

An example of r(class) results would be the stored output from the "tabulation" command. Load the *nhanes* dataset and tabulate the variable entitled race. The *nhanes* dataset is loaded using the command "webuse nhanes2l, clear". The last symbol in the name of the dataset is the letter "l" not the number "1"! Tabulate the variable entitled race. You get a table with the frequencies and percentages for the factor variable. However, Stata retains some parameters in memory that are only replaced when you execute another command, which produces r(class) results when the older results are replaced by the newer results.

You can access the stored results by typing "return list".

```
. tab race

       Race |      Freq.     Percent        Cum.
------------+-----------------------------------
      White |      9,065       87.58       87.58
      Black |      1,086       10.49       98.07
      Other |        200        1.93      100.00
------------+-----------------------------------
      Total |     10,351      100.00

. return list

scalars:
                  r(N) =  10351
                  r(r) =  3
```

r(N) is the total number of observations, and r(r) is the number of levels of the variable being described. You can then use these results in further statistical operations if you wish. You will see an example of this later in the chapter.

Now, for an example of storage of results in e class, regress length on weight from the auto dataset that you previously loaded. The output is reproduced below:

```
. webuse auto, clear
(1978 automobile data)

. regress length weight

      Source |       SS           df       MS      Number of obs   =        74
-------------+----------------------------------   F(1, 72)        =    613.27
       Model |  32389.9843         1  32389.9843   Prob > F        =    0.0000
    Residual |  3802.67784        72    52.81497   R-squared       =    0.8949
-------------+----------------------------------   Adj R-squared   =    0.8935
       Total |  36192.6622        73  495.789893   Root MSE        =    7.2674

------------------------------------------------------------------------------
      length | Coefficient  Std. err.      t    P>|t|     [95% conf. interval]
-------------+----------------------------------------------------------------
      weight |   .0271028   .0010944    24.76   0.000     .0249211    .0292845
       _cons |   106.0965   3.410866    31.11   0.000     99.29708     112.896
------------------------------------------------------------------------------
```

Because the command results in Stata carrying out an inferential analysis, simply typing "return list" will yield a matrix of results.

```
. return list

matrices:
                  r(table) :  9 x 2
```

To see the results of the matrix, we need to save the matrix and then display the results as follows:

```
. matrix a = r(table)

. matrix list a

a[9,2]
            weight       _cons
     b   .02710284   106.09652
    se   .00109443   3.4108659
     t   24.764345   31.105449
pvalue   5.862e-37   1.756e-43
    ll   .02492113    99.29708
    ul   .02928454   112.89595
    df          72          72
  crit   1.9934636   1.9934636
 eform           0           0

.
```

This matrix contains the coefficients for some of the displayed results in the previous estimation command (among other output). However, these results are only held in memory until the next estimation command is issued, so if you want to store them (at least until you close Stata), save them to a matrix as you have just done here.

A more comprehensive list of stored results is accessed in the e() class system and is accessed by issuing "ereturn list". The results for this estimation are shown below. The letter "e" is used to indicate that "estimation" results are stored.

```
. ereturn list

scalars:
                  e(N) =  74
               e(df_m) =  1
               e(df_r) =  72
                  e(F) =  613.2727965692631
                 e(r2) =  .8949323534212077
               e(rmse) =  7.267390862995548
                e(mss) =  32389.98432536247
                e(rss) =  3802.677836799685
               e(r2_a) =  .8934730805520578
                 e(ll) =  -250.7590922914636
               e(ll_0) =  -334.1256749674665
               e(rank) =  2

macros:
            e(cmdline) : "regress length weight"
              e(title) : "Linear regression"
         e(marginsok) : "XB default"
                e(vce) : "ols"
             e(depvar) : "length"
                e(cmd) : "regress"
         e(properties) : "b V"
            e(predict) : "regres_p"
              e(model) : "ols"
          e(estat_cmd) : "regress_estat"

matrices:
                  e(b) :  1 x 2
                  e(V) :  2 x 2
               e(beta) :  1 x 1

functions:
             e(sample)

.
```

VI. SEEDS

Stata's random-number generation functions (for example, runiform() and rnormal() – which generate observations that are from the uniform and standard normal distributions, respectively) do not produce truly random instances. These functions use algorithms and are in fact pseudorandom. The sequences that are produced are determined by a "seed" that is just a number which Stata uses in the generation process. By default, Stata uses the number 123456789 as the default seed every time it is launched. This means that Stata will produce identical results each time you create observations using these random number generators. For this reason, it is usual practice to set a seed at the beginning of each simulation so that identical results are obtained and the analyses are replicable each time you reproduce them.

It's not important which number you use for a seed, but there shouldn't be any pattern to a seed, nor should you set the seed too often in a session.

VII. DEVELOPING A SIMPLE PROGRAM

Let's develop another program.

First of all, create a variable x which has a random normal distribution with a mean of 4 and a standard deviation of 3. This is done by using the inbuilt command rnormal() in Stata which creates a normal distribution with a mean of 0 and a standard deviation of 1. To get a distribution with a mean of 4 and a standard deviation of 3, you will need to multiply the normal distribution which is created by using rnormal() by the constant 3 and then add the number 4. Start with an empty dataset. Assume this dataset will contain 1,000 observations. Once the observations are added, summarise the dataset. This is accomplished by the following code:

```
. clear

. set obs 1000
Number of observations (_N) was 0, now 1,000.

. gen x = (rnormal() *3) + 4

. summ x

    Variable |        Obs        Mean    Std. dev.       Min        Max
-------------+---------------------------------------------------------
           x |      1,000     4.03767    2.916568  -4.971561    15.5703

.
```

As the generation of the observations is a stochastic process, the mean and standard deviation are not exactly what was specified. However, we would expect that if we repeated this process 1,000 times, we would end up with results that were closer to the real values specified in the creation of the variable.

There are several ways to accomplish this. You could create this process 1,000 times and export the results to a Stata temporary file and then summarise the results using a loop.

However, you could simply create a program that creates the dataset 1,000 times and uses Stata's inbuilt package "simulate", which will do the above for you seamlessly.

To make the results replicable, it is desirable that you set a seed.

This program creates 1000 datasets, each of which contains 1,000 observations from a normal distribution with a mean of 4 and a standard deviation of 3. This is done by invoking the Stata command of rnormal(), multiplying the output by 3 and then adding 4. The next step is to summarise the data that has been generated. The summarise command will store the values for mean and standard deviation for each of the 1000 datasets in values that are assigned to the r class. It is now necessary to save these values to scalars (which can be named, for convenience, mean and sd). These values need to be the returned output from the program now being created and will be stored in a dataset which is created by Stata to hold the output of the simulations. Assign the name mean_-normal to this program. The name is chosen so that it is unlikely to clash with previously defined command which already exists in Stata. An example of a program file which achieves this output is shown below.

```
capture program drop mean_normal
program mean_normal, rclass
drop _all
set obs 1000
gen x = (3* rnormal()) + 4
summ x
return scalar mean = r(mean)
return scalar sd = r(sd)
end

simulate mean = r(mean) sd = r(sd), reps(1000): mean_normal seed
(32743)
```

Once the program has run and the dataset has been produced, you can browse the results, which will consist of 1,000 rows of data that contain the values for mean and standard deviation for each of the datasets that were created by the program mean_normal.

To obtain the overall summary values for mean and standard deviation, simply issue the summarise command.

The codes "return scalar mean" and "return scalar sd" are used to save the results to a local macro that is then extracted by the subsequent use of the program "simulate".

CHAPTER 14

Tables of Baseline Characteristics

THE TABLE OF BASELINE CHARACTERISTICS (Table 14.1) is very frequently encountered in statistical reports and in published literature. This table summarises the variables that were used in a study grouped by another variable (the summary variable) which is categorical in nature. If the study were a randomised controlled trial, the summary variable is likely to be the allocated arms of the trial, presented with a final column showing the totals across the rows. For a cohort study, the summary variable is likely to be the levels of the exposure variable. For cross-sectional studies, the summary variable is likely to be the predictor variable. In case-control studies, the summary variable is likely to be the outcome status (cases and controls).

The table of baseline characteristics usually contains summary statistics for the variables that were used in subsequent analyses (usually the confounding variables in the relationship between the predictor and outcome). Looking at Table 14.1 gives the reader a general impression of how well-balanced the arms are and whether or not any results obtained may be due to imbalances between the arms. In the past, statistical tests were performed (and reported) for Table 14.1, showing the *p* value of the test that attempted to identify imbalances between the arms of the dataset. Although some journals continue to report *p* values in Table 14.1, this practice is not usually followed in clinical trials today. The tables that will be demonstrated in this chapter will not contain *p* values.

DOI: 10.1201/9781003483779-14

TABLE 14.1 Table of Baseline Characteristics

	Sex					
	Male N = 4,915 (47.5%)		Female N = 5,436 (52.5%)		Total N = 10,351 (100%)	
	Mean	(sd)	Mean	(sd)	Mean	(sd)
Hematocrit (%)	44.10	(3.09)	40.07	(3.06)	41.99	(3.67)
Age (years)	47.42	(17.17)	47.72	(17.26)	47.58	(17.21)
	Median	(IQR)	Median	(IQR)	Median	(IQR)
Height (cm)	174.60	(9.30)	161.20	(8.90)	167.30	(14.10)
Systolic blood pressure	130.00	(24.00)	124.00	(30.00)	128.00	(28.00)
	n	(%)	n	(%)	n	(%)
Region						
NE	1,018	(20.71)	1,078	(19.83)	2,096	(20.25)
MW	1,310	(26.65)	1,464	(26.93)	2,774	(26.80)
S	1,332	(27.10)	1,521	(27.98)	2,853	(27.56)
W	1,255	(25.53)	1,373	(25.26)	2,628	(25.39)

Table 14.1 is an example of the distributions of several variables that are taken from the previously encountered Second National Health and Nutrition Examination Survey dataset.. You can load this dataset with the Stata command "webuse nhanes2l, clear" (the final character in the name of the dataset is the letter "l" not the number "1").

There are several packages that can produce similar tables in Stata, but the underlying code is explained in this section. It is helpful to review the underlying code so that subsequent (more complicated tables) can be produced (for example, a table that displays the output from statistical testing).

Ultimately, coding for the production of statistical tables ensures that the output is reliably produced (a very important aspect of data analysis in clinical trials). Once you are able to produce tables efficiently using only coding, you can then automate the production of the entire report (which is more time-efficient than making the tables and entering them into the subsequent report manually).

Stata (first introduced in version 18) uses a suite of interlinked commands to enable automation of reports, but perhaps the two most important commands to consider are "table" and "collect". "table" can accommodate many different types of layouts and is flexible enough to allow you to define and amend the characteristics of rows and columns and even produce separate tables by the levels of a grouping variable.

Stata's table command basically specifies the following syntax for producing tables:

table ([row]) ([column]) ([table (by)])

I. TABLE OF MEAN AND STANDARD DEVIATION BY A CATEGORICAL VARIABLE

Load the nhanes dataset (webuse nhanes2l, clear) which you have already encountered. The aim is to provide the mean and standard deviation of iron for each region in the dataset.

The first layout gives mean and standard deviation as column headings for the regions which are displayed as rows.

```
. table (region), stat(mean iron) stat(sd iron)
```

	Mean	Standard deviation
Region		
NE	99.72567	32.65621
MW	99.7801	34.46851
S	96.68735	34.37376
W	101.8649	34.27908
Total	99.44595	34.08279

This layout is not ideal, as if you wanted to add more variables for the summary statistics, the table would need to expand horizontally, not vertically (which is the usual format). The better code lists the summary measures horizontally:

```
. table () (region), stat(mean iron) stat(sd iron)
```

	Region				
	NE	MW	S	W	Total
Mean	99.72567	99.7801	96.68735	101.8649	99.44595
Standard deviation	32.65621	34.46851	34.37376	34.27908	34.08279

This output format is much better than that which was produced in the first table because if you wanted to list the median and interquartile range, you would simply add those to the table command and they would appear at the bottom of the table. The statistic p50 means the 50th centile (the median), and the statistic iqr refers to the interquartile range.

```
. table () (region), stat(mean iron) stat(sd iron) stat(p50 iron) stat(iqr iron)
```

	Region				
	NE	MW	S	W	Total
Mean	99.72567	99.7801	96.68735	101.8649	99.44595
Standard deviation	32.65621	34.46851	34.37376	34.27908	34.08279
50th percentile	96	95	93	98	95
Interquartile range	41	42	44	46	44

What if the results from the table above were required for two variables? Currently, the statistics produced are only related to the variable iron. For example, the table command listed below would produce a table of these results for both iron as well as hematocrit results (the variable name in the dataset is hct).

```
. table () (region), stat(mean iron hct) stat(sd iron hct) ///
> stat(p50 iron hct) stat(iqr iron hct)
```

	Region				
	NE	MW	S	W	Total
Mean					
Serum iron (mcg/dL)	99.72567	99.7801	96.68735	101.8649	99.44595
Hematocrit (%)	42.12281	41.88951	41.88941	42.0855	41.98648
Standard deviation					
Serum iron (mcg/dL)	32.65621	34.46851	34.37376	34.27908	34.08279
Hematocrit (%)	3.532943	3.6085	3.882322	3.614539	3.67368
50th percentile					
Serum iron (mcg/dL)	96	95	93	98	95
Hematocrit (%)	42	42	42	42	42
Interquartile range					
Serum iron (mcg/dL)	41	42	44	46	44
Hematocrit (%)	5	5	5.299999	5	5

The table above now groups the variables within the statistical parameters (so that each of the four statistical parameters has two levels – iron and hematocrit). It is desirable to have all the statistical output for each variable grouped together. When Stata makes a table, it retains information about the table in the form of "dimensions". To access these data, issue the command "collect dims", and the following appears:

```
. collect dims

Collection dimensions
Collection: Table
-----------------------------------------------
                         Dimension   No. levels
-----------------------------------------------
Layout, style, header, label
                            cmdset   1
                           colname   2
                           command   1
                            region   5
                            result   4
                           statcmd   4
                               var   2

Style only
                      border_block   4
                         cell_type   4
-----------------------------------------------
```

Within the output, there are five levels for region and four levels for result.

To find out what data these levels contain:

```
. collect levelsof region

Collection: Table
 Dimension: region
    Levels: 1 2 3 4 .m
```

The variable region has four levels:

```
. tab region

     Region |      Freq.     Percent        Cum.
------------+-----------------------------------
         NE |      2,096       20.25       20.25
         MW |      2,774       26.80       47.05
          S |      2,853       27.56       74.61
          W |      2,628       25.39      100.00
------------+-----------------------------------
      Total |     10,351      100.00
```

The numbers 1 to 4 from the command "collect levelsof region" correspond to the levels of regions NE, MW, S and W, respectively. The fifth level (.m) refers to the column containing the values for "total". This level does not exist within the dataset but is added by Stata when it creates a table.

The four levels of result are unsurprisingly the statistical parameters of mean, median, iqr and standard deviation.

```
. collect levelsof result

Collection: Table
 Dimension: result
    Levels: iqr mean p50 sd
```

The command "layout" is used to rearrange the table that we obtained above so that we can reorganise the rows into the primary grouping variable being the variable name and the statistical parameters being grouped within variables. The symbol (#) is used to denote that the statistical parameters are grouped within the variables.

```
. collect layout (colname#result) (region)

Collection: Table
      Rows: colname#result
   Columns: region
   Table 1: 10 x 5
```

	Region				
	NE	MW	S	W	Total
Serum iron (mcg/dL)					
Mean	99.72567	99.7801	96.68735	101.8649	99.44595
Standard deviation	32.65621	34.46851	34.37376	34.27908	34.08279
50th percentile	96	95	93	98	95
Interquartile range	41	42	44	46	44
Hematocrit (%)					
Mean	42.12281	41.88951	41.88941	42.0855	41.98648
Standard deviation	3.532943	3.6085	3.882322	3.614539	3.67368
50th percentile	42	42	42	42	42
Interquartile range	5	5	5.299999	5	5

To produce a series of tables of statistical output (i.e. summary statistics grouped within each variable) with each level of region having its own table:

A more usually encountered table (output truncated to fit page) ...

```
. collect layout (colname#result) () (region)

Collection: Table
      Rows: colname#result
    Tables: region
   Table 1: 10 x 1
   Table 2: 10 x 1
   Table 3: 10 x 1
   Table 4: 10 x 1
   Table 5: 10 x 1

Region = NE

--------------------------------------------
Serum iron (mcg/dL)          |
  Mean                       |     99.72567
  Standard deviation         |     32.65621
  50th percentile            |           96
  Interquartile range        |           41
Hematocrit (%)               |
  Mean                       |     42.12281
  Standard deviation         |     3.532943
  50th percentile            |           42
  Interquartile range        |            5
--------------------------------------------


Region = MW

--------------------------------------------
Serum iron (mcg/dL)          |
  Mean                       |      99.7801
  Standard deviation         |     34.46851
  50th percentile            |           95
  Interquartile range        |           42
Hematocrit (%)               |
  Mean                       |     41.88951
  Standard deviation         |       3.6085
  50th percentile            |           42
  Interquartile range        |            5
--------------------------------------------


Region = S

--------------------------------------------
Serum iron (mcg/dL)          |
  Mean                       |     96.68735
  Standard deviation         |     34.37376
  50th percentile            |           93
  Interquartile range        |           44
Hematocrit (%)               |
  Mean                       |     41.88941
```

The next table will display the mean and standard deviation for a series of variables by sex:

```
. table () (sex) (), stat(mean iron hct hgb tibc) stat(sd iron hct hgb tibc)
```

	Sex		
	Male	Female	Total
Mean			
Serum iron (mcg/dL)	103.6798	95.61792	99.44595
Hematocrit (%)	44.10391	40.072	41.98648
Hemoglobin (g/dL)	15.07042	13.52809	14.26044
Total iron bind. cap. (mcg/dL)	359.9166	373.3779	366.986
Standard deviation			
Serum iron (mcg/dL)	33.82182	33.86747	34.08279
Hematocrit (%)	3.085013	3.061896	3.67368
Hemoglobin (g/dL)	1.169799	1.133243	1.384677
Total iron bind. cap. (mcg/dL)	50.828	58.93811	55.64079

It is more common, however, for the means and standard deviations to be displayed on the same row. To achieve this, the means and standard deviations need to be recoded so that for each level of sex (i.e. male, female and total), the mean and standard deviation will appear. That means the table will have six columns.

```
. collect layout (colname) (sex#result[mean sd])

Collection: Table
      Rows: colname
   Columns: sex#result[mean sd]
   Table 1: 4 x 6
```

	Sex					
	Male		Female		Total	
	Mean	Standard deviation	Mean	Standard deviation	Mean	Standard deviation
Serum iron (mcg/dL)	103.6798	33.82182	95.61792	33.86747	99.44595	34.08279
Hematocrit (%)	44.10391	3.085013	40.072	3.061896	41.98648	3.67368
Hemoglobin (g/dL)	15.07042	1.169799	13.52809	1.133243	14.26044	1.384677
Total iron bind. cap. (mcg/dL)	359.9166	50.828	373.3779	58.93811	366.986	55.64079

To change the output format from four decimal places to two decimal places:

```
. collect style cell result, nformat(%9.2fc)

.
. collect preview
```

	Sex					
	Male		Female		Total	
	Mean	Standard deviation	Mean	Standard deviation	Mean	Standard deviation
Serum iron (mcg/dL)	103.68	33.82	95.62	33.87	99.45	34.08
Hematocrit (%)	44.10	3.09	40.07	3.06	41.99	3.67
Hemoglobin (g/dL)	15.07	1.17	13.53	1.13	14.26	1.38
Total iron bind. cap. (mcg/dL)	359.92	50.83	373.38	58.94	366.99	55.64

To put brackets around the figures in the column labelled "Standard deviation":

```
. collect style cell result[sd], sformat("(%s%%)")

. collect preview
```

	Sex					
	Male		Female		Total	
	Mean	Standard deviation	Mean	Standard deviation	Mean	Standard deviation
Serum iron (mcg/dL)	103.68	(33.82%)	95.62	(33.87%)	99.45	(34.08%)
Hematocrit (%)	44.10	(3.09%)	40.07	(3.06%)	41.99	(3.67%)
Hemoglobin (g/dL)	15.07	(1.17%)	13.53	(1.13%)	14.26	(1.38%)
Total iron bind. cap. (mcg/dL)	359.92	(50.83%)	373.38	(58.94%)	366.99	(55.64%)

To change the name of the heading "Standard deviation" to "sd":

```
. collect label levels result sd "sd", modify

. collect preview
```

	Sex					
	Male		Female		Total	
	Mean	sd	Mean	sd	Mean	sd
Serum iron (mcg/dL)	103.68	(33.82%)	95.62	(33.87%)	99.45	(34.08%)
Hematocrit (%)	44.10	(3.09%)	40.07	(3.06%)	41.99	(3.67%)
Hemoglobin (g/dL)	15.07	(1.17%)	13.53	(1.13%)	14.26	(1.38%)
Total iron bind. cap. (mcg/dL)	359.92	(50.83%)	373.38	(58.94%)	366.99	(55.64%)

The next step is to add a title:

```
. collect title "Table 1: Mean and sd for baseline variables"

. collect preview
```

Table 1: Mean and sd for baseline variables

	Sex					
	Male		Female		Total	
	Mean	sd	Mean	sd	Mean	sd
Serum iron (mcg/dL)	103.68	(33.82%)	95.62	(33.87%)	99.45	(34.08%)
Hematocrit (%)	44.10	(3.09%)	40.07	(3.06%)	41.99	(3.67%)
Hemoglobin (g/dL)	15.07	(1.17%)	13.53	(1.13%)	14.26	(1.38%)
Total iron bind. cap. (mcg/dL)	359.92	(50.83%)	373.38	(58.94%)	366.99	(55.64%)

To ensure that the table displays appropriately on the page when it is exported to a Word document, issue the following command: "collect style putdocx, layout(autofitcontents)".

Finally, export the table to a Word document named "Table_1.doc", replacing any previously produced table if one exists on disc. The file that is produced is saved in the working directory using the following command:

"collect export "Table_1.docx", replace as(docx)

So far, the table produced has only had one type of data (i.e. continuous normally distributed). To add categorical variables to the table (e.g. race and region), start by producing the basic table again:

```
. table () (sex) (), stat(mean iron hct hgb tibc) stat(sd iron hct hgb tibc) ///
> stat(fvfrequency race region) stat(fvpercent race region)
```

	Sex		
	Male	Female	Total
Mean			
Serum iron (mcg/dL)	103.6798	95.61792	99.44595
Hematocrit (%)	44.10391	40.072	41.98648
Hemoglobin (g/dL)	15.07042	13.52809	14.26044
Total iron bind. cap. (mcg/dL)	359.9166	373.3779	366.986
Standard deviation			
Serum iron (mcg/dL)	33.82182	33.86747	34.08279
Hematocrit (%)	3.085013	3.061896	3.67368
Hemoglobin (g/dL)	1.169799	1.133243	1.384677
Total iron bind. cap. (mcg/dL)	50.828	58.93811	55.64079
Factor-variable frequency			
Race=White	4,312	4,753	9,065
Race=Black	500	586	1,086
Race=Other	103	97	200
Region=NE	1,018	1,078	2,096
Region=MW	1,310	1,464	2,774
Region=S	1,332	1,521	2,853
Region=W	1,255	1,373	2,628
Factor-variable percent			
Race=White	87.73	87.44	87.58
Race=Black	10.17	10.78	10.49
Race=Other	2.10	1.78	1.93
Region=NE	20.71	19.83	20.25
Region=MW	26.65	26.93	26.80
Region=S	27.10	27.98	27.56
Region=W	25.53	25.26	25.39

Again, it is necessary to reorganise the table so that frequencies are next to percentages and means next to standard deviations. In this case, it's easier to create a new column (1) which will contain the results of both means and frequencies and column (2) which will contain the results of both standard deviations as well as percentages.

To achieve this, we recode the results and then change the layout format as below:

```
.
. collect recode result `"mean"' = `"1"' `"sd"' = `"2"' ///
> `"fvfrequency"' = `"1"' `"fvpercent"' = `"2"'
(66 items recoded in collection Table)

.
. collect layout (colname) (sex#result[1 2])

Collection: Table
      Rows: colname
   Columns: sex#result[1 2]
   Table 1: 11 x 6
```

	Sex					
	Male		Female		Total	
	1	2	1	2	1	2
Serum iron (mcg/dL)	103.6798	33.82182	95.61792	33.86747	99.44595	34.08279
Hematocrit (%)	44.10391	3.085013	40.072	3.061896	41.98648	3.67368
Hemoglobin (g/dL)	15.07042	1.169799	13.52809	1.133243	14.26044	1.384677
Total iron bind. cap. (mcg/dL)	359.9166	50.828	373.3779	58.93811	366.986	55.64079
Race=White	4312	87.73143	4753	87.43561	9065	87.57608
Race=Black	500	10.17294	586	10.77999	1086	10.49174
Race=Other	103	2.095626	97	1.7844	200	1.93218
Region=NE	1018	20.71211	1078	19.83076	2096	20.24925
Region=MW	1310	26.6531	1464	26.93157	2774	26.79934
Region=S	1332	27.10071	1521	27.98013	2853	27.56255
Region=W	1255	25.53408	1373	25.25754	2628	25.38885

To change the number of decimal places to 2 for the mean and standard deviation of the continuous variables and also for the percentages of the continuous variables:

```
. collect style cell result[2] colname[iron hct hgb tibc]#result[1], nformat(%9.2fc)

.
. collect preview
```

	Sex					
	Male		Female		Total	
	1	2	1	2	1	2
Serum iron (mcg/dL)	103.68	33.82	95.62	33.87	99.45	34.08
Hematocrit (%)	44.10	3.09	40.07	3.06	41.99	3.67
Hemoglobin (g/dL)	15.07	1.17	13.53	1.13	14.26	1.38
Total iron bind. cap. (mcg/dL)	359.92	50.83	373.38	58.94	366.99	55.64
Race=White	4312	87.73	4753	87.44	9065	87.58
Race=Black	500	10.17	586	10.78	1086	10.49
Race=Other	103	2.10	97	1.78	200	1.93
Region=NE	1018	20.71	1078	19.83	2096	20.25
Region=MW	1310	26.65	1464	26.93	2774	26.80
Region=S	1332	27.10	1521	27.98	2853	27.56
Region=W	1255	25.53	1373	25.26	2628	25.39

To add parentheses for the percentage and standard deviation columns as well as percentage signs for the categorical variables:

```
. collect style cell colname[iron hct hgb tibc]#result[2], sformat("(%s)")

. collect style cell colname[race region]#result[2], sformat("(%s%%)")

.
. collect preview
```

	Sex					
	Male		Female		Total	
	1	2	1	2	1	2
Serum iron (mcg/dL)	103.68	(33.82)	95.62	(33.87)	99.45	(34.08)
Hematocrit (%)	44.10	(3.09)	40.07	(3.06)	41.99	(3.67)
Hemoglobin (g/dL)	15.07	(1.17)	13.53	(1.13)	14.26	(1.38)
Total iron bind. cap. (mcg/dL)	359.92	(50.83)	373.38	(58.94)	366.99	(55.64)
Race=White	4312	(87.73%)	4753	(87.44%)	9065	(87.58%)
Race=Black	500	(10.17%)	586	(10.78%)	1086	(10.49%)
Race=Other	103	(2.10%)	97	(1.78%)	200	(1.93%)
Region=NE	1018	(20.71%)	1078	(19.83%)	2096	(20.25%)
Region=MW	1310	(26.65%)	1464	(26.93%)	2774	(26.80%)
Region=S	1332	(27.10%)	1521	(27.98%)	2853	(27.56%)
Region=W	1255	(25.53%)	1373	(25.26%)	2628	(25.39%)

To remove the column headings of 1 and 2:

```
. collect style header result, level(hide)

.
. collect preview
```

	Sex					
	Male		Female		Total	
Serum iron (mcg/dL)	103.68	(33.82)	95.62	(33.87)	99.45	(34.08)
Hematocrit (%)	44.10	(3.09)	40.07	(3.06)	41.99	(3.67)
Hemoglobin (g/dL)	15.07	(1.17)	13.53	(1.13)	14.26	(1.38)
Total iron bind. cap. (mcg/dL)	359.92	(50.83)	373.38	(58.94)	366.99	(55.64)
Race=White	4312	(87.73%)	4753	(87.44%)	9065	(87.58%)
Race=Black	500	(10.17%)	586	(10.78%)	1086	(10.49%)
Race=Other	103	(2.10%)	97	(1.78%)	200	(1.93%)
Region=NE	1018	(20.71%)	1078	(19.83%)	2096	(20.25%)
Region=MW	1310	(26.65%)	1464	(26.93%)	2774	(26.80%)
Region=S	1332	(27.10%)	1521	(27.98%)	2853	(27.56%)
Region=W	1255	(25.53%)	1373	(25.26%)	2628	(25.39%)

To remove the "=" from the labels of the categorical variables and to reorganise the levels so that they lie under a grouping name:

```
. collect style row stack, nobinder indent spacer

.

.

. collect preview
```

	Sex					
	Male		Female		Total	
Serum iron (mcg/dL)	103.68	(33.82)	95.62	(33.87)	99.45	(34.08)
Hematocrit (%)	44.10	(3.09)	40.07	(3.06)	41.99	(3.67)
Hemoglobin (g/dL)	15.07	(1.17)	13.53	(1.13)	14.26	(1.38)
Total iron bind. cap. (mcg/dL)	359.92	50.83	373.38	58.94	366.99	55.64
Race						
White	4312	(87.73%)	4753	(87.44%)	9065	(87.58%)
Black	500	(10.17%)	586	(10.78%)	1086	(10.49%)
Other	103	(2.10%)	97	(1.78%)	200	(1.93%)
Region						
NE	1018	(20.71%)	1078	(19.83%)	2096	(20.25%)
MW	1310	(26.65%)	1464	(26.93%)	2774	(26.80%)
S	1332	(27.10%)	1521	(27.98%)	2853	(27.56%)
W	1255	(25.53%)	1373	(25.26%)	2628	(25.39%)

The next step is to add the number of participants in each column heading of the grouping variable sex (i.e. the total number of participants who were male, female and overall).

The first step is to contract the dataset so that you have the number and percentages for each level of sex:

"contract sex, freq(n) percent(p)"

Then generate a label that contains these data for each level:

gen label = "N = " +string(n, "%9.0fc") + " (" + string(p, "%9.1fc") + "%)"

The command string(n, "%9.0fc") is taking the number found in the variable name n (which was created when the dataset was contracted) and applying the format of %9.0fc (means no decimal places as these are integers).

Finally, create new labels with these data. The commands "preserve" and "restore" and placed before and after the contract command and the generation of the labels for males and females so that the original data are not replaced. The label for.m (which represents the total column in the table) is generated by counting the number of non-missing values of sex and then generating a label using this value.

```
. * Contracting the data and generating labels for males and females
. preserve

. qui contract sex, freq(n) percent(p)

. gen label = "N = " +string(n , "%9.0fc") + " (" + string(p, "%9.1fc") + "%)"

. local male_label = label[1]

.
. local female_label = label[2]

. restore

. * Generating label for total
. count if sex !=.
  10,351

. local total = "N = " +string(`r(N)', "%9.0fc") + " (100%)"

. display "`total'"
N = 10,351 (100%)

. * Applying labels
. collect label levels sex 1 "Male `male_label'" 2 "Female `female_label'" .m "Total `total'", modify

. collect preview
```

	Sex					
	Male N = 4,915 (47.5%)		Female N = 5,436 (52.5%)		Total N = 10,351 (100%)	
Serum iron (mcg/dL)	103.68	(33.82)	95.62	(33.87)	99.45	(34.08)
Hematocrit (%)	44.10	(3.09)	40.07	(3.06)	41.99	(3.67)
Hemoglobin (g/dL)	15.07	(1.17)	13.53	(1.13)	14.26	(1.38)
Total iron bind. cap. (mcg/dL)	359.92	50.83	373.38	58.94	366.99	55.64
Race						
White	4312	(87.73%)	4753	(87.44%)	9065	(87.58%)
Black	500	(10.17%)	586	(10.78%)	1086	(10.49%)
Other	103	(2.10%)	97	(1.78%)	200	(1.93%)
Region						
NE	1018	(20.71%)	1078	(19.83%)	2096	(20.25%)
MW	1310	(26.65%)	1464	(26.93%)	2774	(26.80%)
S	1332	(27.10%)	1521	(27.98%)	2853	(27.56%)
W	1255	(25.53%)	1373	(25.26%)	2628	(25.39%)

It is necessary to create rows that indicate which results are mean (sd) and which are N (%) as well as an empty row that becomes a spacer to separate rows where necessary with blank rows. To achieve this, the collect get command is used. This command is usually used to obtain coefficients from estimation commands, but it is being reused in this context to place the necessary headings in the table. The rest of the code in this snippet formats the headers and aligns the output, etc.

```
.         qui collect get _r_b1 = " ", tags(sex[1] colname[empty])

.         levelsof sex, local(levels_by_var)
1 2

.         local levels_by_var `levels_by_var' .m

.         foreach i of local levels_by_var{
  2.         qui collect get _r_b2 = "n", tags(sex[`i'] colname[name1])
  3.         qui collect get _r_b3 = "(%)", tags(sex[`i'] colname[name1])
  4.         qui collect get _r_b4 = "Mean", tags(sex[`i'] colname[name2])
  5.         qui collect get _r_b5 = "(sd)", tags(sex[`i'] colname[name2])
  6.         }

.
.         qui collect recode result `"_r_b2"' = `"1"' ///
>                                                    `"_r_b3"' = `"2"' ///
>                                                    `"_r_b4"' = `"1"' ///
>                                                    `"_r_b5"' = `"2"'      ///
>                                                    `"_r_b1"' = `"1"'

.         qui collect style cell cell_type[column-header], font(, size(11) bold)

.         qui collect style cell colname[name1 name2 name3], font(, bold)

.         qui collect style cell result[2], halign(left)

.         collect layout (colname[name2 iron hct hgb tibc empty name1 race region]) (sex#result[1 2])

Collection: Table
      Rows: colname[name2 iron hct hgb tibc empty name1 race region]
   Columns: sex#result[1 2]
   Table 1: 18 x 6

-----------------------------------------------------------------------------------------------------------
                                  |                                     Sex
                                  |   Male N = 4,915 (47.5%)   Female N = 5,436 (52.5%)   Total N = 10,351 (100%)
----------------------------------+------------------------------------------------------------------------
name2                             |      Mean   (sd)                Mean   (sd)                 Mean   (sd)
Serum iron (mcg/dL)               |    103.68   (33.82)            95.62   (33.87)              99.45   (34.08)
Hematocrit (%)                    |     44.10   (3.09)             40.07   (3.06)               41.99   (3.67)
Hemoglobin (g/dL)                 |     15.07   (1.17)             13.53   (1.13)               14.26   (1.38)
Total iron bind. cap. (mcg/dL)    |    359.92   50.83             373.38   58.94               366.99   55.64
empty                             |
name1                             |         n   (%)                    n   (%)                      n   (%)
                                  |
Race                              |
  White                           |      4312   (87.73%)            4753   (87.44%)              9065   (87.58%)
  Black                           |       500   (10.17%)             586   (10.78%)              1086   (10.49%)
```

The final step is to remove the column names for the headers we just created for the table.

```
.         ****************************
.         ** Formatting Final Table **
.         ****************************
.         qui collect style header colname[empty], level(hide)

.         qui collect style header colname[name1], level(hide)

.         qui collect style header colname[name2], level(hide)

.
.         collect preview
```

	Sex					
	Male N = 4,915 (47.5%)		Female N = 5,436 (52.5%)		Total N = 10,351 (100%)	
	Mean	(sd)	Mean	(sd)	Mean	(sd)
Serum iron (mcg/dL)	103.68	(33.82)	95.62	(33.87)	99.45	(34.08)
Hematocrit (%)	44.10	(3.09)	40.07	(3.06)	41.99	(3.67)
Hemoglobin (g/dL)	15.07	(1.17)	13.53	(1.13)	14.26	(1.38)
Total iron bind. cap. (mcg/dL)	359.92	50.83	373.38	58.94	366.99	55.64
	n	(%)	n	(%)	n	(%)
Race						
White	4312	(87.73%)	4753	(87.44%)	9065	(87.58%)
Black	500	(10.17%)	586	(10.78%)	1086	(10.49%)
Other	103	(2.10%)	97	(1.78%)	200	(1.93%)
Region						
NE	1018	(20.71%)	1078	(19.83%)	2096	(20.25%)
MW	1310	(26.65%)	1464	(26.93%)	2774	(26.80%)
S	1332	(27.10%)	1521	(27.98%)	2853	(27.56%)
W	1255	(25.53%)	1373	(25.26%)	2628	(25.39%)

CHAPTER 15

Automated Reporting

I. INTRODUCTION

The generation of automated reports is highly desirable because doing so not only is more time-efficient that when tables and reports are produced individually, but also the reproducibility of the results is increased as there are fewer (if any) opportunities for errors to be introduced (apart from the obvious errors in the code). Some methods of producing tables include copying results from the Stata screen or log files into manually created tables in a Word processing document (or exporting the results to an interim Excel file and then reimporting them to Microsoft Word). This chapter describes the production of reports directly from Stata to a Word document.

II. PUTDOCX

The command suite of "putdocx" is the interface between Microsoft Word and Stata. The first step in producing an automated report is to first produce the individual images, plots, charts and tables that you want to include in the report and to save these objects. In the case of tables, these can be exported using "collect export", which will create a file with extension .stjson. The other objects can be exported using .jpg, .pdf, etc.

Once you have produced the components of the report, it is now time to import these into a report and format the report (including a front page, headers, page numbers, etc.).

"putdocx clear" closes any previously opened documents. "putdocx begin" begins the document (which is built in memory). Usually, a

DOI: 10.1201/9781003483779-15

document will have a front page, which will not have a page number, header or footer. Then there is the body of the document which follows. When you create a new document using the "putdocx begin" command, the footers and headings you will use on the subsequent pages are also created at the same time. It is helpful to create two types of headers and two types of footers. The code below shows that the first header and footer have the sub-option "first", which indicates that these will be applied to the first page of the document and so should not contain page numbers.

```
putdocx clear
putdocx begin, footer(firstfooter, first) ///
header(firstheader, first) header(bodyheader)
footer(bodyfooter)
```

Since the header and footer for the first page will, for this example, contain no information, they do not need further attention. The footer and header for the body of the text need to be formatted, and text, page numbers, etc., need to be added.

a. Header

To add the text "Clinical Trials Unit" to the header, have it aligned to the centre of the page and format the text in Calibri font size 12 (black) using the following code:

```
* Header
putdocx paragraph, toheader(bodyheader) halign(center)
font(Calibri, 12, black)
putdocx text ("Clinical Trials Unit")
```

b. footer

To add the text "CTU Trial" to the middle bottom of the page using a font size 12 in red, use the commands indicated below. You can also use the additional two lines of code at the end to add page numbers in bold to the footer.

```
* Footer
putdocx paragraph, tofooter(bodyfooter) halign(center)
font(Calibri, 12, red)
putdocx text ("CTU Trial")
putdocx paragraph, tofooter(bodyfooter)
putdocx pagenumber, bold
```

c. Front Page

All of the commands thus far have been used to create and format the text, which will appear in the header and footer for the main body text. The next step is to add text to the first page itself.

```
putdocx paragraph, halign(center) font(Calibri, 18, black)
putdocx text ("Sample Report"), bold
putdocx paragraph
putdocx paragraph
putdocx paragraph, style(Heading2) halign(center)
putdocx text ("Prepared by John Smith")
putdocx pagebreak
```

d. Subsequent Pages

The command "putdocx image" followed by the location of the image will insert an image you have into the page.

The following code will insert a heading of the default style "Heading 2" into the page with the text "Table 1" in black followed by a page break.

```
putdocx paragraph, style(Heading2) font(Calibri, 12, black)
putdocx text ("Table 1")
putdocx pagebreak
```

e. Placing Previously Produced Tables into the Document

Having previously prepared a table and exported it using the command "collect export", it is possible to now import the table into the Word document by using these commands followed by saving the final document.

```
collect use " … ./table_1", replace
putdocx collect
putdocx pagebreak
putdocx save "Sample_Report.docx", replace
```

CHAPTER 16

pretty_suite Packages for Easy Tables

I. INTRODUCTION

As you see, the coding for the production of tables of baseline characteristics (or any tables where the output is grouped by a categorical variable) can be tricky. Luckily there is an .ado file that vastly simplifies this process. The package is named "pretty_baseline" and is installed using the "ssc install" commands. To install the package, issue this command to Stata:

```
ssc install pretty_suite
```

One of the installed pacakges is named "pretty_baseline" and makes pretty tables of baseline characteristics. The second package to be installed is called "pretty_logistic" and makes pretty output for automated reporting when using logistic regression.

If you have previously installed this package, it's a very good idea to update your .ado files that you have downloaded from the web from time to time. This is done by issuing the following command:

```
ado update, update
Load the nhanes dataset
webuse nhanes2l, clear
```


DOI: 10.1201/9781003483779-16

The package pretty_baseline is very flexible, and an overview can be obtained by using the helpfiles that have been installed with the package using the following command:

```
help pretty_baseline
```

pretty_baseline generates a table of baseline characteristics of publication quality. pretty_baseline generates grouped results by any categorical variable with greater than or equal to two groups. It will also produce a table with summary statistics if you omit a grouping variable. If there is missingness in the grouping variable, a column with missing values will be produced. There are four types of data that are accommodated. Normally distributed continuous variables, continuous variables with a skewed distribution, categorical and count variables. The default number of decimal places for all statistics for continuous data is two decimal places after the decimal point. For categorical and count data, the counts and percentages are shown. The percentage output has a default of one decimal place.

The default variable labels for the table are the value labels from the dataset. Where value labels are not specified, variable names will be presented.

If you do not use a grouping "by" variable, then the package gives you only totals for each subset of the variables. The other options available are shown in the help file. The notation used to specify the options includes some letters in CAPITALS and some letters in lowercase. This terminology is used to indicate that the letters in capitals can be used for each of the given options if you wish to abbreviate them. Alternatively, you can use all of the letters. Irrespective of whether or not you abbreviate, the options in Stata commands are in lowercase.

i. Using the option "CONTNormal" will produce data by group summarised by mean and standard deviation.

ii. The option CONTSkewed will produce output summarised by median and interquartile range values (IQR).

iii. The option CATEGorical will produce frequency and percentages for the specified variables and will handle both counts as well as categorical variables.

iv. The option FCONT specifies the format for continuous variables.

v. The option FCATEG specified the format categorical and/or count variables.

vi. The option TITLE allows you to specify a title for the table.

vii. The option SAVing allows you to export the table as a Word document to disk.

viii. The option POSition allows you to specify the vertical sequence in which the categories of data are displayed in your table. The default is categorical, followed by continuous normal and then continuous skewed data.

ix. The option REPLACE indicates that you wish to replace a previously saved version that you have exported with the current version of the table.

The options are explored in the following series of tables:

1. Table with only grouping variable

```
. * Grouping Variable Only - Table 1
.          pretty_baseline, ///
>          by(sex) ///
>          title("Table 1: Grouping Variable Only"
(4 items recoded in collection Table)

Table 1: Grouping Variable Only
-------------------------------------------
                   Sex
       Male                  Female
   N          (%)       N           (%)
-------------------------------------------
4915    (47.48%)    5436    (52.52%)
-------------------------------------------

.        qui collect save "table_1", replace
```

2. Table with variables which are continuous and normally distributed

```
. * Continuous normal - Table 2
.         pretty_baseline, ///
>         by(sex) ///
>         contn(bp*) ///
>         title("Table 2: Continuous Normal")
```

Table 2: Continuous Normal

	Sex					
	Male N = 4,915 (47.5%)		Female N = 5,436 (52.5%)		Total N = 10,351 (100%)	
	Mean	(sd)	Mean	(sd)	Mean	(sd)
Systolic blood pressure	132.89	(20.99)	129.07	(25.13)	130.88	(23.33)
Diastolic blood pressure	83.45	(12.58)	80.15	(13.04)	81.72	(12.93)

```
.         qui collect save "table_2", replace
```

3. Table with variables which are continuous with skewed distributions

```
. * Continuous skewed - Table 3
.         pretty_baseline, ///
>         by(sex) ///
>         conts(lead) ///
>         title("Table 3: Continuous Skewed")
```

Table 3: Continuous Skewed

	Sex					
	Male N = 4,915 (47.5%)		Female N = 5,436 (52.5%)		Total N = 10,351 (100%)	
	Median	(IQR)	Median	(IQR)	Median	(IQR)
Lead (mcg/dL)	16.00	(8.00)	11.00	(5.00)	13.00	(7.00)

```
.         qui collect save "table_3", replace
```

4. Table with a categorical variable

```
. * Categorical variable - Table 4
.         pretty_baseline, ///
>         by(sex) ///
>         categ(race) ///
>         title("Table 4: Categorical Variable")
```

Table 4: Categorical Variable

	Sex					
	Male N = 4,915 (47.5%)		Female N = 5,436 (52.5%)		Total N = 10,351 (100%)	
	n	(%)	n	(%)	n	(%)
Race						
Black	499	(10.15)	582	(10.71)	1,081	(10.44)
Other	103	(2.10)	97	(1.78)	200	(1.93)
White	4,302	(87.53)	4,747	(87.33)	9,049	(87.42)
Missing	11	(0.22)	10	(0.18)	21	(0.20)

```
.         qui collect save "table_4", replace
```

5. Table with a count variable

```
. * Count numeric variable - Table 5
.         pretty_baseline, ///
>         by(sex) ///
>         categ(hsizgp) ///
>         title("Table 5: Count Variable ")

Table 5: Count Variable
```

	Sex					
	Male N = 4,915 (47.5%)		Female N = 5,436 (52.5%)		Total N = 10,351 (100%)	
	n	(%)	n	(%)	n	(%)
# in household or 5 if #>=5						
1	672	(13.67)	1,057	(19.44)	1,729	(16.70)
2	1,802	(36.66)	1,828	(33.63)	3,630	(35.07)
3	843	(17.15)	899	(16.54)	1,742	(16.83)
4	786	(15.99)	790	(14.53)	1,576	(15.23)
Missing	812	(16.52)	862	(15.86)	1,674	(16.17)

```
.         qui collect save "table_5", replace
```

6. Table produced using abbreviated variable names

```
. ** Abbreviated Variable Names - Table 6
.         pretty_baseline, ///
>         by(se) ///
>         contn(bpsy) ///
>         categ(reg) ///
>         conts(bm) ///
>         title("Table 6: Abbreviated variable names")

Table 6: Abbreviated Variable Names
```

	Sex					
	Male N = 4,915 (47.5%)		Female N = 5,436 (52.5%)		Total N = 10,351 (100%)	
	Mean	(sd)	Mean	(sd)	Mean	(sd)
Systolic blood pressure	132.89	(20.99)	129.07	(25.13)	130.88	(23.33)
	Median	(IQR)	Median	(IQR)	Median	(IQR)
Body mass index (BMI)	25.15	(4.98)	24.42	(6.77)	24.82	(5.88)
	n	(%)	n	(%)	n	(%)
Region						
NE	1,018	(20.71)	1,078	(19.83)	2,096	(20.25)
MW	1,310	(26.65)	1,464	(26.93)	2,774	(26.80)
S	1,332	(27.10)	1,521	(27.98)	2,853	(27.56)
W	1,255	(25.53)	1,373	(25.26)	2,628	(25.39)

```
.         qui collect save "table_6", replace
```

7. Table in which the vertical layout of the categories of data are specified

```
. ** Specified layout - Table 7
.         pretty_baseline, ///
>         by(se) ///
>         categ(reg) ///
>         contn(bp*) ///
>         conts(bm) ///
>         position(categ contn conts) ///
>         title("Table 7: Specified layout")
```

Table 7: Specified Layout

	Sex					
	Male N = 4,915 (47.5%)		Female N = 5,436 (52.5%)		Total N = 10,351 (100%)	
	n	(%)	n	(%)	n	(%)
Region						
NE	1,018	(20.71)	1,078	(19.83)	2,096	(20.25)
MW	1,310	(26.65)	1,464	(26.93)	2,774	(26.80)
S	1,332	(27.10)	1,521	(27.98)	2,853	(27.56)
W	1,255	(25.53)	1,373	(25.26)	2,628	(25.39)
	Mean	(sd)	Mean	(sd)	Mean	(sd)
Systolic blood pressure	132.89	(20.99)	129.07	(25.13)	130.88	(23.33)
Diastolic blood pressure	83.45	(12.58)	80.15	(13.04)	81.72	(12.93)
	Median	(IQR)	Median	(IQR)	Median	(IQR)
Body mass index (BMI)	25.15	(4.98)	24.42	(6.77)	24.82	(5.88)

```
.         qui collect save "table_7", replace
```

8. Table in which the output format is changed

```
. ** Formatting  - Table 8
. ** continuous changed to 4 dp and categorical frequencies to 2 dp
.         pretty_baseline, ///
>         by(sex) ///
>         categ(region) ///
>         contn(bp*) ///
>         conts(bmi) ///
>         position(categ contn conts) ///
>         fcont(%9.4fc) ///
>         fcateg(%9.2fc) ///
>         title("Table 8: formatting of output")
```

Table 8: Formatting of Output

	Sex					
	Male N = 4,915 (47.5%)		Female N = 5,436 (52.5%)		Total N = 10,351 (100%)	
	n	(%)	n	(%)	n	(%)
Region						
NE	1,018	(20.71)	1,078	(19.83)	2,096	(20.25)
MW	1,310	(26.65)	1,464	(26.93)	2,774	(26.80)
S	1,332	(27.10)	1,521	(27.98)	2,853	(27.56)
W	1,255	(25.53)	1,373	(25.26)	2,628	(25.39)
	Mean	(sd)	Mean	(sd)	Mean	(sd)
Systolic blood pressure	132.8877	(20.9927)	129.0679	(25.1268)	130.8817	(23.3327)
Diastolic blood pressure	83.4482	(12.5826)	80.1479	(13.0353)	81.7150	(12.9272)
	Median	(IQR)	Median	(IQR)	Median	(IQR)
Body mass index (BMI)	25.1490	(4.9781)	24.4197	(6.7688)	24.8181	(5.8847)

```
.         qui collect save "table_8", replace
```

9. Table with "if/in" specifications

```
. ** if / in - Table 9
.         pretty_baseline if zinc <100 in 1/10000, ///
>         by(sex) ///
>         categ(region) ///
>         contn(bp*) ///
>         conts(bmi) ///
>         position(categ contn conts) ///
>         fcont(%9.4fc) ///
>         fcateg(%9.2fc) ///
>         title("Table 9: Table using if and in") ///
>         replace
```

Table 9: Table Using if and in

	Sex					
	Male N = 3,248 (43.8%)		Female N = 4,167 (56.2%)		Total N = 7,415 (100%)	
	n	(%)	n	(%)	n	(%)
Region						
NE	749	(23.06)	927	(22.25)	1,676	(22.60)
MW	737	(22.69)	985	(23.64)	1,722	(23.22)
S	956	(29.43)	1,250	(30.00)	2,206	(29.75)
W	806	(24.82)	1,005	(24.12)	1,811	(24.42)
	Mean	(sd)	Mean	(sd)	Mean	(sd)
Systolic blood pressure	133.7460	(21.1311)	129.2985	(25.1403)	131.2467	(23.5706)
Diastolic blood pressure	83.8217	(12.5655)	80.2083	(12.9615)	81.7911	(12.9138)
	Median	(IQR)	Median	(IQR)	Median	(IQR)
Body mass index (BMI)	25.1061	(5.0847)	24.3854	(6.5746)	24.7454	(5.8764)

```
.         qui collect save "table_9", replace
```

10. Table without frequency weights (for comparison with Table 11)

```
.
. ** fweight -1 - Table 10
.         pretty_baseline, ///
>         by(sex) ///
>         categ(region) ///
>         contn(bp*) conts(bmi) ///
>         position(categ contn conts) ///
>         fcont(%9.4fc) ///
>         fcateg(%9.2fc) ///
>         title("Table 10: Table without fweights") ///
>         replace
```

Table 10: Table Without Fweights

	Sex					
	Male N = 4,915 (47.5%)		Female N = 5,436 (52.5%)		Total N = 10,351 (100%)	
	n	(%)	n	(%)	n	(%)
Region						
NE	1,018	(20.71)	1,078	(19.83)	2,096	(20.25)
MW	1,310	(26.65)	1,464	(26.93)	2,774	(26.80)
S	1,332	(27.10)	1,521	(27.98)	2,853	(27.56)
W	1,255	(25.53)	1,373	(25.26)	2,628	(25.39)
	Mean	(sd)	Mean	(sd)	Mean	(sd)
Systolic blood pressure	132.8877	(20.9927)	129.0679	(25.1268)	130.8817	(23.3327)
Diastolic blood pressure	83.4482	(12.5826)	80.1479	(13.0353)	81.7150	(12.9272)
	Median	(IQR)	Median	(IQR)	Median	(IQR)
Body mass index (BMI)	25.1490	(4.9781)	24.4197	(6.7688)	24.8181	(5.8847)

```
.         qui collect save "table_10", replace
```

11. Table with frequency weights applied

```
.
. ** fweight - 2 - Table 11
.         pretty_baseline [fweight = 2], ///
>         by(sex) ///
>         categ(region) ///
>         contn(bp*) conts(bmi) ///
>         position(categ contn conts) ///
>         fcont(%9.4fc) ///
>         fcateg(%9.2fc) ///
>         title("Table 11: Table with fweights") ///
>         replace
```

Table 11: Table With Fweights

	Sex					
	Male N = 9,830 (47.5%)		Female N = 10,872 (52.5%)		Total N = 20,702 (100%)	
	n	(%)	n	(%)	n	(%)
Region						
NE	2,036	(20.71)	2,156	(19.83)	4,192	(20.25)
MW	2,620	(26.65)	2,928	(26.93)	5,548	(26.80)
S	2,664	(27.10)	3,042	(27.98)	5,706	(27.56)
W	2,510	(25.53)	2,746	(25.26)	5,256	(25.39)
	Mean	(sd)	Mean	(sd)	Mean	(sd)
Systolic blood pressure	132.8877	(20.9917)	129.0679	(25.1257)	130.8817	(23.3321)
Diastolic blood pressure	83.4482	(12.5820)	80.1479	(13.0347)	81.7150	(12.9269)
	Median	(IQR)	Median	(IQR)	Median	(IQR)
Body mass index (BMI)	25.1490	(4.9781)	24.4197	(6.7688)	24.8181	(5.8847)

```
.         qui collect save "table_11", replace
.
```

Verify that the numbers in each level of the categorical variable are double those in Table 10.

CHAPTER 17

Tables with Output from Statistical Tests

THE PREVIOUS CHAPTERS have reviewed how to make tables of descriptive statistics. This chapter will introduce how to make specialised tables of output from statistical tests. These tables can also be saved and used in the process of making automated reports.

This chapter will present a series of tables and the code needed to produce them. Once these techniques are mastered, it is more likely that other more specialised tables could then be attempted.

1. TABLE OF RESULTS FROM A LOGISTIC REGRESSION

This is an example of a table that would be used to report the results of a logistic regression analysis. In this case, using the nhanes dataset, the following table reports the odds ratio of having heart attack (binary outcome) with sex as a predictor. The results are shown here:

Table 2: Logistic regression of Heart Attack by Sex

	Total number	Number affected	Odds	(95% CI)	Std. error	p-value
Male	4,915	318	1		0	
Female	5,436	158	0.433	(0.356 to 0.526)	0.043	<0.001

DOI: 10.1201/9781003483779-17

The steps for obtaining this table are shown below.

The Stata subcommand "command" for the table command is now used. The coefficients are listed before the logistic command so that Stata knows which values you wish to use to make the table.

```
. table, command(_r_b _r_lb _r_ub _r_se _r_p: logistic heartatk i.sex) nformat(%9.3fc)

------------------------------
Coefficient         |
  Sex=Male          |   1.000
  Sex=Female        |   0.433
  Intercept         |   0.069
95% lower bound     |
  Sex=Female        |   0.356
  Intercept         |   0.062
95% upper bound     |
  Sex=Female        |   0.526
  Intercept         |   0.078
Std. error          |
  Sex=Male          |   0.000
  Sex=Female        |   0.043
  Intercept         |   0.004
p-value             |
  Sex=Female        |   0.000
  Intercept         |   0.000
------------------------------
```

The next step is to use the "layout" command to change the layout to one that is horizontal rather than vertical.

```
. collect layout (colname) (result[ _r_b _r_lb _r_ub _r_se _r_p])

Collection: Table
      Rows: colname
   Columns: result[ _r_b _r_lb _r_ub _r_se _r_p]
   Table 1: 3 x 5
```

	Coefficient	95% lower bound	95% upper bound	Std. error	p-value
Sex=Male	1.000			0.000	
Sex=Female	0.433	0.356	0.526	0.043	0.000
Intercept	0.069	0.062	0.078	0.004	0.000

The values for the total number of participants in each category of sex and the number affected in each category now need to be obtained, extracted and placed into the results table just obtained.

Tabulate the outcome with the predictor to obtain the values required.

```
.
. tabulate heartatk sex

   Prior heart |          Sex
        attack |      Male     Female |     Total
---------------+----------------------+----------
 No heart attack |    4,597      5,276 |     9,873
Had heart attack |      318        158 |       476
---------------+----------------------+----------
         Total |    4,915      5,434 |    10,349
```

You can obtain the four figures you need using the "collect get" command. You need to let Stata know that these figures will be placed in the table of results by providing each number with a unique name beginning with _r (a system of nomenclature used by Stata). The subcommand "tags" is used to specify the column heading, and the tag "colname" is used to specify the row name. Those results that relate to "males" will be tagged "1.sex", and those results that relate to "females" will be tagged "2.sex". The column with "totals" is therefore tagged with total[1], and the column that shows the number of participants who had the outcome is tagged total[2].

```
.
.       count if sex == 1
  4,915

.       collect get _r_mt = `r(N)', tags(total[1] colname[1.sex])

.
.       count if sex == 2
  5,436

.       collect get _r_ft = `r(N)', tags(total[1] colname[2.sex])

.
.       count if sex ==1 & heartatk == 1
  318

.       collect get _r_ma = `r(N)', tags(total[2] colname[1.sex])

.
.       count if sex ==2 & heartatk == 1
  158

.       collect get _r_fa = `r(N)', tags(total[2] colname[2.sex])

.
.       collect layout (colname) (total result[ _r_b _r_lb _r_ub _r_se _r_p])

Collection: Table
      Rows: colname
   Columns: total result[ _r_b _r_lb _r_ub _r_se _r_p]
   Table 1: 3 x 7
```

	total 1	total 2	Coefficient	95% lower bound	95% upper bound	Std. error	p-value
Sex=Male	4,915.000	318.000	1.000			0.000	
Sex=Female	5,436.000	158.000	0.433	0.356	0.526	0.043	0.000
Intercept			0.069	0.062	0.078	0.004	0.000

Currently the upper and lower boundaries for the 95% confidence intervals appear in two separate columns when it is preferable that they be presented as one statistic. This is achieved by creating a single statistic named combined_ci in which the upper and lower values are concatenated, separated by the word "to" and excess space is trimmed off.

```
.
. **      Concatenating upper and lower boundaries
.         collect composite define combined_ci = _r_lb _r_ub, delimiter(" to ") replace trim

.         collect layout (colname) (total result[ _r_b combined_ci _r_se _r_p])

Collection: Table
      Rows: colname
   Columns: total result[ _r_b combined_ci _r_se _r_p]
   Table 1: 3 x 6
```

	total 1	2	Coefficient	95% lower bound to 95% upper bound	Std. error	p-value
Sex=Male	4,915.000	318.000	1.000		0.000	
Sex=Female	5,436.000	158.000	0.433	0.356 to 0.526	0.043	0.000
Intercept			0.069	0.062 to 0.078	0.004	0.000

The code to remove the heading "total" and provide the other column headings with sensible titles is:

```
.
.         collect style header total, title(hide)

.
.
.         collect label levels total 1 "Total number" 2 "Number affected", modify

.         collect label levels result combined_ci "95% CI"

.         collect label levels result _r_b "Odds", modify

.
.         collect preview
```

	Total number	Number affected	Odds	95% CI	Std. error	p-value
Sex=Male	4,915.000	318.000	1.000		0.000	
Sex=Female	5,436.000	158.000	0.433	0.356 to 0.526	0.043	0.000
Intercept			0.069	0.062 to 0.078	0.004	0.000

The code to format the output and change the *p* value from 0.000 to <0.001 is shown below:

```
.
. collect style cell total, nformat(%9.0fc)

. collect style cell result[_r_b]#colname[1.sex], nformat(%9.0fc)

. collect style cell result[_r_se]#colname[1.sex], nformat(%9.0fc)

.
. collect style row stack, nobinder indent

. collect style header sex, title(hide)

.
. collect style cell result[combined_ci], sformat("(%s)")

.
. collect style cell result[_r_p], min(0.001, label("<0.001"))

.
. collect preview
```

	Total number	Number affected	Odds	(95% CI)	Std. error	p-value
Male	4,915	318	1		0	
Female	5,436	158	0.433	(0.356 to 0.526)	0.043	<0.001
Intercept			0.069	(0.062 to 0.078)	0.004	<0.001

Finally, the code to add a title and remove the intercept is shown below. You can now choose to export this collection and then use the table in an automated report, or you can export the table to a Word document, .pdf, etc.

```
. ** Title of Table
.         collect title "Table 2: Logistic regression of Heart Attack by Sex"

.
. ** Removing Intercept from results
.         collect layout (colname[1.sex 2.sex]) (total result[_r_b combined_ci _r_se _r_p])

Collection: Table
      Rows: colname[1.sex 2.sex]
   Columns: total result[_r_b combined_ci _r_se _r_p]
   Table 1: 2 x 6

Table 2: Logistic regression of Heart Attack by Sex
```

	Total number	Number affected	Odds	(95% CI)	Std. error	p-value
Male	4,915	318	1		0	
Female	5,436	158	0.433	(0.356 to 0.526)	0.043	<0.001

An alternative would be to use the automated package "pretty_logistic" which was installed when you downloaded "pretty_suite". The packages allows output in odds ratios, risk ratios and risk differences. As usual, you can save the file and import into an automated report.

```
.
. pretty_logistic, predictor(sex) outcome(heartatk) log("or")

Collection: Table
      Rows: colname[1.sex 2.sex]
   Columns: total result[_r_b combined_ci _r_se _r_p]
   Table 1: 3 x 6
```

	Total number	Number affected	Odds	(95% CI)	Std. error	p-value
Sex						
Male	4,915	318	1		0	
Female	5,436	158	0.433	(0.356 to0.526)	0.043	<0.001

FIGURE 17.1

2. TABLE AND GRAPH FROM A SURVIVAL ANALYSIS

This table presents results from a cox regression model of survival data. The table to be produced is:

	HR	95%CI	SE	p-Value
Intervention				
Placebo	1		0	
Active	0.133	0.056 to 0.314	0.058	<0.001

Download data from the Stata website and change the labels for the variable encoding data for the drug. These data are already set for survival analysis when they are downloaded.

```
use https://www.stata-press.com/data/r18/drugtr.dta, clear
label define drug 0 "Placebo" 1 "Active", replace
label values drug drug
label variable drug "Intervention"
```

The first command to make the table simply lists the coefficients of interest with the stcox command:

```
.
. table, command(_r_b _r_lb _r_ub _r_p: stcox i.drug)

--------------------------------------------
Coefficient                     |
  Intervention=Placebo          |          1
  Intervention=Active           |   .1327581
95% lower bound                 |
  Intervention=Active           |   .0560555
95% upper bound                 |
  Intervention=Active           |   .3144157
p-value                         |
  Intervention=Active           |      0.000
--------------------------------------------

.
```

The next command changes the layout of the table from vertical to horizontal.

```
.       collect layout (colname) (result)

Collection: Table
      Rows: colname
   Columns: result
   Table 1: 2 x 4

----------------------------------------------------------------------------------------
                     |  Coefficient   95% lower bound   95% upper bound   p-value
---------------------+------------------------------------------------------------------
Intervention=Placebo |            1
Intervention=Active  |     .1327581          .0560555          .3144157     0.000
----------------------------------------------------------------------------------------
```

The next set of commands then formats the table (these commands have mostly been previously encountered).

```
.       collect label levels result _r_b "HR" combined_ci "95%CI" _r_se "SE" _r_p "p-Value", modify

.       collect style cell result, nformat(%9.3fc)

.       collect style cell colname[0.drug]#result, nformat(%9.0f)

.       collect style cell result[_r_p], min(0.001, label("<0.001"))

.       collect style row stack, nobinder indent spacer

.
.       collect preview

-------------------------------------------------------
             |     HR            95%CI     SE   p-Value
-------------+-----------------------------------------
Intervention |
  Placebo    |      1                       0
  Active     |  0.133   0.056 to 0.314  0.058    <0.001
-------------------------------------------------------
```

The next suite of commands produces the Cumulative Hazard graph and exports it as a .png object so that it can be subsequently imported into an automated report.

```
sts graph, cumhaz by(drug) title("") xtitle("Months to Death") ///
ytitle("Cumulative Hazard") ///
legend(order(1 "Control" 2 "Treatment")) ///
risktable(, size(small) order(1 "Control" 2 "Treatment"))
graph export "km.png", replace
```

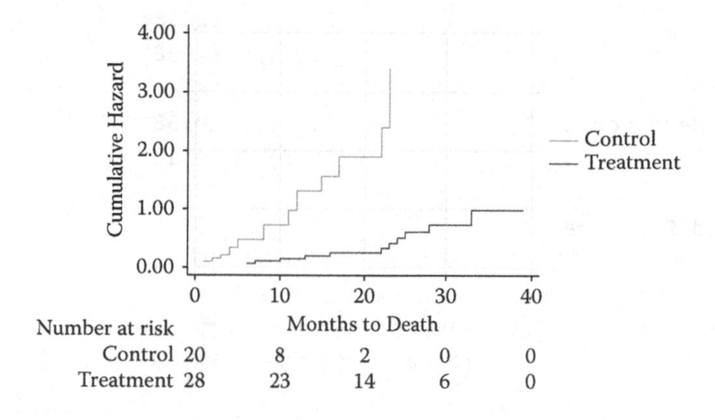

3. TABLE OF MULTIPLE REGRESSION RESULTS

This table presents the results of multiple regression analyses in a format that allows relatively easy comparison of the coefficients.

This table is patterned on a webinar by Stata, which demonstrated the production of a similar table and on which this code is largely based.

	(1)	(2)	(3)
Black	3.19	4.23	0.58
	(0.75)	(0.75)	(0.53)
Other	-1.83	-1.71	-2.46
	(1.67)	(1.65)	(1.15)
Hematocrit (%)		-0.09	-0.20
		(0.11)	(0.07)
Female		-52.52	-24.86
		(6.27)	(4.38)
Female x Hematocrit (%)		1.21	0.58
		(0.15)	(0.10)
High Blood Pressure=1			33.81
			(0.32)
Intercept	130.58	136.52	125.69
	(0.24)	(4.75)	(3.32)
AIC	94568	94387	86954
BIC	94590	94430	87005

To create this table, start by downloading the data from the web, changing the variable label for the variable that encodes for high blood pressure, and clearing the memory that holds data on the collect command.

```
webuse nhanes2l, clear
label variable highbp “High Blood Pressure”
collect clear
```

The next step is to fit the three models and collect the coefficients.

```
** MODEL ONE
collect get _r_b _r_se, tag(model[(1)]): regress bpsystol i.race
collect get AIC=r(S)[1,“AIC”] BIC=r(S)[1,“BIC”], tag(model[(1)]): estat ic
```

```
** MODEL TWO
collect get _r_b _r_se, tag(model[(2)]): regress bpsystol i.race
c.hct##i.sex
collect get AIC=r(S)[1,"AIC"] BIC=r(S)[1,"BIC"], tag(model[(2)]): estat ic

// MODEL 3
collect get _r_b _r_se, tag(model[(3)]): regress bpsystol i.race
c.hct##i.sex i.highbp
collect get AIC=r(S)[1,"AIC"] BIC=r(S)[1,"BIC"], tag(model[(3)]): estat ic
```

Next, make the table using the now-familiar layout command.

```
. collect layout (colname#result) (model)

Collection: default
      Rows: colname#result
   Columns: model
   Table 1: 19 x 3
```

	(1)	(2)	(3)
Black	3.19	4.23	0.58
	(0.75)	(0.75)	(0.53)
Other	-1.83	-1.71	-2.46
	(1.67)	(1.65)	(1.15)
Hematocrit (%)		-0.09	-0.20
		(0.11)	(0.07)
Female		-52.52	-24.86
		(6.27)	(4.38)
Female x Hematocrit (%)		1.21	0.58
		(0.15)	(0.10)
High Blood Pressure=1			33.81
			(0.32)
Intercept	130.58	136.52	125.69
	(0.24)	(4.75)	(3.32)

Remove the vertical line to the left of the results.

```
. collect style cell border_block, border(right, pattern(nil))

. collect preview

-------------------------------------------------------
                              (1)       (2)       (3)
-------------------------------------------------------
Black                        3.19      4.23      0.58
                           (0.75)    (0.75)    (0.53)
Other                       -1.83     -1.71     -2.46
                           (1.67)    (1.65)    (1.15)

Hematocrit (%)                        -0.09     -0.20
                                     (0.11)    (0.07)

Female                               -52.52    -24.86
                                     (6.27)    (4.38)

Female x Hematocrit (%)                1.21      0.58
                                     (0.15)    (0.10)

High Blood Pressure=1                           33.81
                                               (0.32)

Intercept                  130.58    136.52    125.69
                           (0.24)    (4.75)    (3.32)
-------------------------------------------------------
```

The next set of commands formats the display and puts parentheses on the standard errors.

```
. collect style cell, nformat(%5.2f)

. collect style cell result[_r_se], sformat("(%s)")

. collect preview
```

	(1)	(2)	(3)
Black	3.19	4.23	0.58
	(0.75)	(0.75)	(0.53)
Other	-1.83	-1.71	-2.46
	(1.67)	(1.65)	(1.15)
Hematocrit (%)		-0.09	-0.20
		(0.11)	(0.07)
Female		-52.52	-24.86
		(6.27)	(4.38)
Female x Hematocrit (%)		1.21	0.58
		(0.15)	(0.10)
High Blood Pressure=1			33.81
			(0.32)
Intercept	130.58	136.52	125.69
	(0.24)	(4.75)	(3.32)

The final steps are to remove the result headers of "coefficient" and "std. error", replace the "#" symbol with "x", add an extra space between columns to increase readability and add in the results for AIC and BIC.

```
. collect style header result, level(hide)

. collect style column, extraspace(1)

. collect style row stack, spacer delimiter(" x ")

. collect style header result[AIC BIC], level(label)

. collect style cell result[AIC BIC], nformat(%8.0f)

. collect layout (colname#result result[AIC BIC]) (model)

Collection: default
      Rows: colname#result result[AIC BIC]
   Columns: model
   Table 1: 23 x 3

----------------------------------------------------
                              (1)      (2)      (3)
----------------------------------------------------
Black                        3.19     4.23     0.58
                           (0.75)   (0.75)   (0.53)
Other                       -1.83    -1.71    -2.46
                           (1.67)   (1.65)   (1.15)

Hematocrit (%)                       -0.09    -0.20
                                    (0.11)   (0.07)

Female                              -52.52   -24.86
                                    (6.27)   (4.38)

Female x Hematocrit (%)               1.21     0.58
                                    (0.15)   (0.10)

High Blood Pressure=1                         33.81
                                             (0.32)

Intercept                  130.58   136.52   125.69
                           (0.24)   (4.75)   (3.32)

AIC                         94568    94387    86954

BIC                         94590    94430    87005
----------------------------------------------------
```

You can now export either the collection or the table itself for use later.

Index

Printed in the United States
by Baker & Taylor Publisher Services

Printed in the United States
by Baker & Taylor Publisher Services